LIVING WITH
LEWY BODY DEMENTIA

ONE CAREGIVER'S PERSONAL,
IN-DEPTH EXPERIENCE

JUDY TOWNE
JENNINGS PT, MA

WESTBOW
PRESS
A DIVISION OF THOMAS NELSON

ISBN: 978-1-4497-6096-0 (e)
ISBN: 978-1-4497-6095-3 (sc)
ISBN: 978-1-4497-6094-6 (hc)
Library of Congress Control Number: 2012913668

WestBow Press books may be ordered through booksellers or by contacting:

WestBow Press
A Division of Thomas Nelson
1663 Liberty Drive
Bloomington, IN 47403
www.westbowpress.com
1-(866) 928-1240

Printed in the United States of America
WestBow Press rev. date: 09/04/2012

**The Author is a Professional Physical Therapist with
Many Years Experience With Movement Disorders**

The information that I presented is believed to be accurate based on personal and professional experience of author with references up to date at the time of writing.

Any activities or suggestions are assumed at the risk of the reader. Medical consultations should determine specific individual activities. Author welcomes any reader to report any misinformation.

Acknowledgements

Bob Houston, an accomplished editor, who taught me to write with
clarity, conciseness, and commas.
Peter and Linda Towne, who advised me on how and what
to include from the perspective of a physical therapist,
with honor for Dean as a beloved brother-in-law.
For all the kind people who were willing to read
the book and offer their suggestions.
It is a better work because of the collective wisdom that has been offered.

To my loving husband, Dean, who taught me the power of humor.

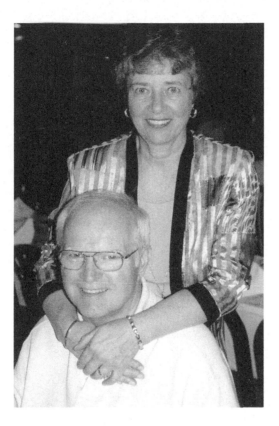

Contents

KEY IDEA: Lewy Body Dementia has many of the same symptoms as Parkinson disease in addition to mental symptoms similar to Alzheimer's disease. Unlike both PD and Alzheimer's, symptoms wax and wane. The important point of this chapter is to understand the particulars of all three diseases. How are they similar and how are they different.

KEY IDEA: The attitudes of a caregiver and the sick spouse are critically important. Without the effort to stay positive, any serious disease can eat away at self esteem, confidence, and the joy of living. If those involved can develop an "adventure attitude"; the days, weeks, months, and years within the disease experience can prove meaningful. An adventure attitude is accepting the hand that is dealt, expecting to win.

KEY IDEA: Having fun takes work. Organizing both big and little events can make a huge difference in how a person facing a serious illness can maintain mental alertness and physical independence. Events on the calendar do not need to be expensive to be something one can eagerly anticipate.

KEY IDEA: LBD is a multifaceted disease that can cause periods of severe debilitation. During times of heavy stress, the caregiver can reach a point when he or she feels that caregiving is too difficult. Stress overload can occur, often called burn out. It is important to recognize when other options are needed. It does no good for a caregiver to become so overtaxed that he or she is no longer able to provide caregiving services in a positive manner. Many options to relieve burn out are discussed.

KEY IDEA: Walking is Very Important. Maintaining the ability to walk and transfer easily from bed to chair helps foster independence, and makes the job of caregiving easier. At some point the walking pattern will become abnormal due to losses in coordination and balance. When a person begins to walk with a shuffling of feet, or has difficulty moving the feet forward, evaluations by therapists may help. A physical therapist can teach safe walking with assistive devices to help prevent falling.

KEY IDEA: At some point in the process of the disease, daily care skills will be affected. There are many care tips to help someone remain as independent as possible.

KEY IDEA: Organizing the home early in the disease process will help the caregiver be ready when more assistance is needed.

KEY IDEA: Vision, hearing, balance, touch, smell, and taste can all be affected by the disease. Understanding what the world of someone with LBD feels like, can help the caregiver promote comfort and safety.

KEY IDEA: Besides neurological; digestive, circulatory, pulmonary, skin, urinary, sexual functions can all be affected by the disease. Some of the associated problems can make life miserable until a remedy is found.

KEY IDEA: Many activities can bolster the mental and cognitive functions. Humor is one of the best strategies to relieve stress and promote long term memory.

PREFACE

Who Should Read This Book?

Reportedly, 65 million people were providing some level of caregiving in the United States in 2009.[1] Of those, 10% were providing extensive care at level 5, which is the most demanding level of care.[1] The stress of caregiving is so high at level 5 that it can affect the immune system of the caregiver for at least three years.[1]

One source lists the number of people in the United States with Alzheimer's disease as 4 million. One million of those actually have Lewy Body Dementia.[2] Maria Shriver reported in 2010 that Alzheimer's is an epidemic with 10 million women either afflicted or providing caregiving for someone with Alzheimer's.[3] Some of those listed with Alzheimer's may actually have Lewy Body Dementia. It is not easily diagnosed or identified.

The economics, reported in the above 2009 report, estimated that the value of the free services family caregivers provide was in the range of $375 billion a year. "That is almost twice as much as is actually spent on homecare and nursing home services combined ($158 billion)".[1]

It is not possible from the data to determine if the millions of people with Alzheimer's and Lewy Body Dementia are those people listed in the level 5 skill level category. If they aren't, they should be. I was one of the 65 million and I understand the emotional and financial demands of caring for a husband with dementia 24 hours a day.

This book was written to give caregivers "meat and potatoes" suggestions to make their jobs easier. Little suggestions that work can have a significant impact on the stress level of both the caregiver and the patient (spouse or loved one). The simple act of placing red duct tape on the floor helped my husband transfer more easily from the wheelchair to the leisure chair, eliminating my need to repeatedly issue directions at him.

The book is set up to serve the reader's concerns and needs. The topics can be chosen via the Contents page or the Index. The chapters are written to cover a particular characteristic that might be present in someone with Lewy Body Dementia, Parkinson disease, Alzheimer's disease, or Parkinson-Plus-Syndromes.[4] For instance, Chapter 6 discusses all the different patterns of walking that might develop for someone with LBD or late stage Parkinson disease. Many suggestions are offered to help the caregiver understand the physical symptoms affecting walking abilities. The Index is available for easy reference to topics. A Time Line (appendix 1) details Dean's progression with the stages of the disease.

The book is directed at the disease Lewy Body Dementia; however, much of the material throughout the book is applicable to caregiving for any disease that shuts down physical, mental, and emotional capabilities.

Although the suggestions refer to a wife caring for her husband, the particulars are as appropriate for either gender caregiver. Most of the characteristics describing LBD will be appropriate for either a man or a woman.

This is our story: my caregiving experience for my husband. Other people with LBD may not have all the characteristics of the disease that my husband had, nor progress in his particular way. We felt our story was straightforward because Dean did not have any age related diseases such as diabetes or heart issues to complicate the LBD caregiving.

If the suggestions help other caregivers anywhere, our story will have a larger ripple effect of caring compassion. Help is certainly needed. As I launch into this smorgasbord of suggestions, I am expecting the book to stimulate discussion among readers.

Chapter 1

The Beginning

For everything there is a season and a time for every matter under Heaven:
—Ecclesiastes 3:1 Revised Standard Version

It is easy to see the big picture in hindsight. Being a physical therapist did not prepare me for the assault my husband's declining health had on every aspect of our married lives. Maybe I should have been quicker to evaluate my Dean's stooped posture, weak voice, and shuffling gait. Maybe I should have realized that he had a serious illness the first time that he fell. He was standing across from me on the tennis court. I hit a ball to him as I had done for 35 years. As he twisted to avoid being hit, he slowly fell to the ground like a tree in the woods. I should have recognized his lack of balance. I didn't. I was just like any other wife who never expects a beloved husband to have a serious medical condition; I hid in denial. After Dean fell, it took strong pressure from my brother and sister-in-law (both physical therapists) to get me to schedule a work up at The Mayo Clinic in Florida.[5] The beginning of this saga was in the summer of 2005.

Mayo Clinic is a unique medical center. They are set up to explore a medical condition in an efficient, expeditious manner. Dean saw four specialists, had two MRI's, a sleep study, and a colonoscopy in four days. Although we did not get a definitive reason for his balance problems, many maladies were ruled out. We did get a possible diagnosis of Parkinson disease with a recommendation for physical therapy.

Delivering physical therapy to a stranger is far different than watching the miraculous effects of an effective PT program on a loved one. At my brother's clinic, Dean received a thorough PT evaluation and treatment program that stretched and strengthened all the muscles of his body. After several weeks of therapy, Dean was a new man. He was, indeed, sufficiently able to rejoin his tennis buddies for another season of tennis. Dean was walking more quickly and moving on the tennis court with good balance. I was thrilled that I had my husband back. It appeared as if he had averted any serious medical condition.

If that was the end of the story, there would be no reason for this book. For us, as with millions of other people, Dean's balance issues continued to plague him. By the next summer, he complained that he still felt like he had a bad case of "stumbilitis". At times he would catch his toe if he wasn't paying attention. He said his legs felt heavy and awkward.

This time I scheduled an evaluation at Aring Neurology, nearer our home in Cincinnati.[6] Specialists assured us that Dean needed to begin a drug regimen used to treat Parkinson disease (PD).[7,8] My physical therapy problem solving skills kicked in. If he had PD, so be it. I knew about the exercise routine to keep stiff muscles working. Since PD is often projected to be a slowly degenerating disease, I expected us to grow old together. We might need to make some adjustments, but life would not need to change drastically.

How unpredictable life can be! How little I knew about the REAL problems!

I did not know that Dean had been having severe anxiety attacks during the previous three years. During his last year of working, his short term memory began failing him. He could not remember how to do the engineering computations that had been easy and automatic for him for five decades. He had begun to carry little note pads in his pocket to jot down reminders: things to tell me, things to do at work, reports that he had written. This was prompted when he would do a report one day, only to realize that he had already done that report the day before.

The ten months before he was to retire, anxiety about his job skills was paralyzing his performance. He was sure he was going to make some big mistake that would get him fired. He knew that his memory was failing him, and he didn't know why.

Sleep problems were complicating his ability to do his job. He felt like he had weights on his eyelids. If he wasn't moving, his eyelids would drop and he would doze off. To stay alert at work, he drank caffeine sodas and ate candy bars all day. In the last year that he worked, he put on 35 pounds.

Worry turned from embarrassment to frustration, and finally to outright panic when he was asked to retire two months early. In hind sight, I realized that these were the early symptoms of a disease called Lewy Body Dementia (LBD) which were occurring long before he had any physical symptoms.

Lewy Body Dementia was not well known from 1999 to 2006 when we were trying to get a definitive diagnosis. Until he showed the physical symptoms typical of Parkinson disease (stooped posture, forward head, shuffling walking pattern resulting in falls due to lack of balance), we had no reason to seek medical attention. In fact he was not actually diagnosed with Lewy Body Dementia until two years later in 2008, when he complained to our family doctor that he was seeing things that I refused to believe were there. He was having hallucinations in addition to the physical and mental symptoms. After our doctor recommended that I read the description of symptoms listed on the Lewy Body Dementia Association webpage: http://www.lbda.org,[9] I had to admit that Dean's diagnosis was more serious than Parkinson disease. To my amazement, Dean had every symptom listed. There was no doubt that LBD was the correct diagnosis.

That realization felt like a torpedo piercing my chest. My perception of our life together was exploded. I suddenly understood Dean's panic. We faced many questions and no answers. Nothing in my PT education taught me about a Parkinson disease gone wild.

In my effort to provide quality of life to my husband as he maneuvered through the maze of his LBD, I studied, charted all his medical symptoms regularly in a notebook, explored all of our options for activities he could continue to do, and prayed. I had no caregiving manual to teach us how to help him stay independent. This book is the compilation of the trial and error strategies that we used.

When Dean was dealing with a particular problem, we would work together to creatively come up with a solution. As an example, on some days he needed a bit of help to get into our shower. Our shower had the glass doors that did not give him much of an opening. I took the doors completely off, bought an inexpensive shower rod, curtain and rings. With the curtain, he had a lot of room to get into the shower. I installed a bar by the shower opening which gave him just the help he needed to assure his independence with showering.

Any degenerative disease will work to destroy self respect, dignity, and a sense of peace for not only the patient, but for the caregiver and family. LBD was the hand we were dealt; we needed to play it, expecting to win. What worked for us was assuming an "Adventure Attitude". As we negotiated our way through the onslaught of LBD problems, we also created a memorable story. We took three cruises in five years, two of which were in Europe. We loved to travel and didn't let LBD stop our trips all over the country.

We set a goal to be honest, loving, considerate, and accepting of each other. I am not saying that living with LBD is easy, but with the choice to use a great amount of love, with an even greater amount of humor, we made the most of our days.

Reviewing my years of notes allowed me to see both the successes and the mistakes that my husband and I made. Our successes were impressive; we turned a tragedy into an adventure that left positive memories. We are not super special people. Deciding to fight for quality of life can happen for anyone. My hope is that this story of our adventure will make the path for others a bit wider and less rugged.

a time to keep silence, and a time to speak:
—Ecclesiastes 3:7 RSV

Chapter 2

How Lewy Body Dementia Resembles Parkinson Disease and Alzheimer's Disease

A time to seek
—Ecclesiastes 3:6 RSV

Lewy Body Dementia (LBD) is a disease affecting the brain cells in a section of the brain called the Substantia Nigra. It is similar to the breakdown of cells in Parkinson disease (PD). In LBD, however, brain cells in other parts of the brain can also become diseased. For this reason, a person can demonstrate the physical abnormalities characteristic of PD in addition to the cognitive deficiencies similar to Alzheimer's dementia (AD).[10] When I checked sources during our search to understand my husband's disease [5, 7–13], I found LBD had several labels. For simplicity, in this book I will use the labels as Dean's neurologist, Dr. Andrew Duker, UC Physicians,[6] explained them to me. If significant cognitive changes occur at the same time as or within the first year of when Parkinsonian (motor) symptoms start, the clinical diagnosis is Dementia with Lewy Bodies (DLB). If the cognitive changes occur later (e.g., after the first year), the clinical diagnosis is Parkinson Disease with Dementia (PDD). Some professionals believe PDD and DLB are separate diseases, while others believe they are both on a spectrum of disorders.

This distinction was arbitrary for my husband. Dean had many cognitive early signs before the motor symptoms, but he was able to hide his problems. He did not have the hallucinations until two years after the physical problems manifested. The total spectrum of his decline was only obvious in hindsight.

From a caregiver's perspective, it is important to know several diseases can have movement dysfunctions that mimic typical idiopathic PD. In an article, by Arif Dalvi and Stephen Bloomfield, five Parkinson-plus syndromes are described.[4] The five syndromes are listed in appendix 2.

I surely don't expect caregivers to understand the differences in all these different diseases, but caregivers should be assured that the doctors they chose to manage the disease DO understand the differences.

For this book, LBD will be the classification used whether the condition starts with physical symptoms or mental problems. From my caregiver's perspective, simple is better. The most important thing to understand is LBD and the other four Parkinson-plus diseases do not respond effectively to the medication protocol used for typical PD. Secondly, the dementia of LBD may appear similar to Alzheimer's, but it is different. The doctors also need to know the differences between LBD and AD.

Because the breakdown in brain proteins is similar, PD and LBD are sister diseases. LBD, unfortunately, acts more like the deranged son. Unlike the slow and gentle progression we expected with the Parkinson diagnosis, LBD can be very aggressive and rapidly progressive. Faced with this new diagnosis, I needed to arm myself with knowledge and skill. This was not going to be a growing older gracefully disease.

Dean faced major physical hurdles the year he was diagnosed. Neither of us was prepared for the cognitive declines that followed the next year. Until I realized what Dean was experiencing fit the symptom profile for a very different disease, I was concerned I was doing something wrong in how I was caring for him. I needed a book to explain that LBD acts differently than PD. All our resources explained PD well but glossed over the day-to-day particulars we needed to know about LBD.

One important particular was prognosis. LBD is listed as incurable with an average life expectancy after diagnosis of five to seven years. Both PD and AD have life expectancies averaging 10-20 years after diagnosis.

Medical specialists are working to find a more thorough means for diagnosing classic PD without dementia and the other Parkinson-like diseases. But as yet, there are no laboratory tests or brain scans that can quickly determine if the diagnosis is PD, AD, LBD, or something else.

If I were to repeat this experience, as soon as I heard a diagnosis of PD or AD, I would schedule an evaluation with a neurologist who specializes in movement disorders and Parkinsonian symptoms. I would search medical sites on the Internet and take notes on areas of concern. Oh wait! That is what I did with my husband, and we still experienced many setbacks that could have been avoided if I had known in 2005 what I know today.

LBD and PD Are Treated Differently Medically

When a loved one is diagnosed with LBD, the first thing to understand is how vitally important it is to work with family doctors and/or neurology specialists who are fully up to date on all aspects of LBD. The doctors should have the experience to correctly diagnose LBD, prescribe the best drugs, and quickly recognize any oversensitivity to a prescribed drug.

The treatment of choice for PD, AD, and LBD is an individually prescribed arsenal of drugs to combat the motor deficiencies, with different drugs to help retard the loss of memory and reasoning skills associated with the dementia aspect of these diseases. Caregivers should be aware that some drugs for PD may not be helpful in LBD. The levodopa drugs that work well to decrease the motor complications of typical PD have very little effect on the stumbling of LBD and may increase the presence of hallucinations and nausea.

People with LBD can have severe negative reactions to many drugs including non-prescription products. Some decongestants can increase restlessness or confusion in someone with LBD. Drug reactions and interactions are discussed more fully in Chapter 9. Another source on drugs for LBD is a book by the Whitworths.[14]

Tests to Evaluate Movement Disorders

Rather than restating the generic characteristics particular to LBD that can be found online by searching "Lewy body dementia," I have chosen to describe my husband's progression of symptoms from a caregiver's perspective. A timetable of symptoms is included as appendix 1. Recognizing what is abnormal may be the first big step in helping a loved one. I recommend that the potential caregiver and patient make a list of anything that seems out of the ordinary before the first doctor visit. These observations may be very helpful to the doctors when determining a plan of action.

A neurology assessment tries to uncover the reasons for any abnormal patterns of movement, such as Dean's shuffling walking pattern. Doctors need to observe how well the patient's joints are working, how balanced the patient is while walking, and how fast he can complete certain tasks. This kind of assessment is necessary to determine if a person has a neurological disease and, if so, which one. The following four symptoms were assessed to determine Dean's diagnosis.

Did he have a hand tremor when the hand was at rest? For most people with early-stage PD or LBD, a tremor may be seen only in one hand, but both hands may be affected in later stages. Tremors often occur in the feet as well.

Did Dean have a state of rigidity in the muscles of his arms or legs that made it difficult to bend or straighten those joints? The doctor tested for rigidity by pulling slowly on Dean's relaxed bent arm. The doctor was able to diagnose the presence of rigidity by assessing the amount of resistance he felt when attempting to straighten Dean's arm. When present, rigidity may affect walking, balance, arm swing, and hand function.

A third test checked the amount of coordination Dean had in completing a requested activity. He was asked to rapidly alternate a palm up, palm down motion with his hands. People with PD and LBD are often frustrated by slower than normal movements. This is called bradykinesia (brady = slow, kinesia = movement). It may take excessively long amounts of time to do the simple tasks of buttoning buttons, zipping coats, or getting out of a chair or bed. Dean could begin a coordination task well, but the movements would become jumbled with an extended amount of repetition.

The last functional test checked the amount of instability with balance when standing upright. The doctor pulled backward on Dean's shoulders to see if he could correct his balance, which he was able to do. As the disease progresses, persons with PD or LBD lose their balance and fall backward into the doctor's arms, because the balance mechanisms of the body become seriously dysfunctional.

The balance issue is extremely important. Instability may show itself most clearly in how a person walks. In people with PD and LBD, this is usually a shuffling of the feet. In the later stages, a person becomes unable to turn or change directions quickly. And in the more advanced stage of the disease, a person may fall easily.

This explanation of how Dean was tested applies to initial evaluations for PD or LBD. The deterioration in physical functions is similar for both diseases. Unfortunately, in LBD, the abnormal walking pattern, slow uncoordinated movements, and balance issues become compressed into a much shorter span of time from initial diagnosis to severe disabilities. More information about the progression of Parkinsonism movements and testing can be found under Hohen and Yahr Staging Scale and the Unified Parkinson Disease Rating Scale (UPDRS).[15–16]

Lewy Body Dementia Will Have Specific Symptoms

Dean had problems unusual for PD between 2006 and 2008 that kept me looking for a different diagnosis. An example of a strange complication occurred one summer. Dean would become nauseated whenever he ventured out of our air-conditioned house. Nothing we did seemed to help his overreaction to the heat. We did not determine a reason until we read the symptoms for LBD on the Foundation webpage. Multiple systems in the body can be affected with LBD. Sensitivity to temperature changes was listed.

The following is a brief overview of typical symptoms that help determine a diagnosis of Lewy Body Dementia.

Hallucinations are a classic symptom of LBD.[17] Dean was seeing objects that were not there. He complained of aliens sitting on the end of his bed, or black creatures running across our carpet. They were not scary to him, but the doctor explained that hallucinations could get very serious. We needed to get medication to help.

Dementia must be present in some degree for a diagnosis of LBD. The dementia of Lewy Body disease occurs in a different area of the brain than is known for Alzheimer's disease, but it is a gradual loss of thinking abilities, as it is with AD. This may be apparent with memory loss, problem solving difficulties, or inability to focus. Dean needed to write down everything in little note pads to avoid important ideas slipping away from him.

Waxing and waning of symptoms is unique to LBD. The degree of confusion may fluctuate during the course of a day. Dean had fluctuations in the physical skills also. He might not be able to walk well one day and need my help to prevent falling, but be able to walk stairs with no assistance the next day.

LBD is a complicated disease to diagnose because many other symptoms can present that seem unrelated at first. Dean had numerous problems that looked like individual maladies, but were all part of the LBD picture. These should all be reported to the doctors:

Shallow breathing problems and low voice projection
Temperature regulation, either too hot or too cold
Digestion problems such as nausea or constipation
Urinary, bowel, and sexual problems

Any sudden, unexplained loss of consciousness should be reported. This is explained in detail in Chapter 10. It was a very frustrating problem to deal with.

Sleep issues can be a problem. A person may not be able to sleep deeply at night, but then be extremely sleepy during the day. This is often one of the first signs of LBD, well before the physical and mental problems.[13] It was so for my husband. We did not know to consider it as a symptom. Dean would complain that if he closed his eyes anywhere during the day, he would fall asleep. His eyelids always felt very heavy.

Poor reasoning may be present. Dean was unable to explain his declining work performance. He could only tell me that he felt he was not doing good work, which made no sense to me.

Team Approach

We found that it took a team of medical specialists to work through all of Dean's complexities. This is thoroughly discussed in Chapter 13.

The two of us learned to work as a team on a daily basis. As I developed strategies to fit the problems affecting his daily tasks, he worked hard to follow through with those strategies. When he was successful, all of us on his team were successful.

The next chapters explain all those challenges and strategies in detail: help for the emotional instability, physical challenges, daily activity needs, sensory system involvement, mental complications, and general health concerns. Topics can be selected by choice from the Table of Contents or Index. All problems could be occurring concurrently.

Chapter 3

Understanding the Emotional Challenges

and a time to heal;
—Ecclesiastes 3:3 RSV

The emotional assault is the worst. How does a family move from happiness, memorable vacations, and retirement dreams to life with a monster disease that eats away at a loved family member, one day at a time? No one is immune to the feelings of despair: friends, relatives, co-workers, neighbors. This Chapter 3 is placed at the beginning of all the idea chapters because it is, in my opinion, the most important. It is the master plan. The emotional mindset of both the patient and the caregiver are critical to turning the disease catastrophe into a quality of life adventure. Our attitude choices can make living with LBD tolerable.

Acceptance

Acceptance is the first important action to becoming a caregiver. I am no different than any other caregiver. When my husband began to have minor health setbacks, I fairy-dusted them away. Dean HAD to be fine. He was the emotional rock of the family, my best friend, and my confidante.

It took me two years of denial and wishful thinking before I accepted that Dean was dealing with a very serious disease, and I needed to make it a priority in my life. My first step was accepting the fact that I needed to become a caregiver. I didn't want the job. I was not prepared. It was not convenient. After a long cry on the phone with my son, the denial was gone. I was ready to do battle with a malicious disease attacking someone I loved.

The next step after accepting my role as a caregiver was becoming informed about the enemy. If a caregiver doesn't know what to expect, she can not be prepared. Not being prepared is admitting defeat before even waging a fight. The problem with becoming informed is that we must face the reality of how difficult the battle will be. LBD is a life threatening disease that can prove lethal for our loved ones at some point in the future.

My mom's motto was "Where there is a will, there is a way". It takes hard work to become a caring caregiver. The rest of this chapter will offer suggestions to move the new caregiver from the acceptance decision, away from anger and grief, toward a goal of quality of life. Most importantly, this methodology allows any caregiver to move into the scary position as a life manager. I am not promising that acceptance will be easy, but it will be worth it.

An Adventure Attitude

When faced with major life decisions that are difficult, require hard work, and offer no guarantee of success, I offer this suggestion: assume an adventure attitude. Create a big dream instead of assuming the worse. Shoot for the moon, and be willing to do whatever it takes to get there. Take reasonable risks, but be willing to laugh when the plan doesn't work out as expected. Take reasonable risks and be gracious to anyone who helped make the plan work. My favorite motto was to work toward a BIG goal as if everything depended on us, but have faith that everything depended on God.

The biggest example I can use is the adventure that Dean and I had with his dream to continue playing tennis. He knew that he was having physical problems and had already suffered a broken collar bone after falling on a tennis court in 2005. We had been playing tennis as a couple for thirty-five years. It was his favorite sport, and he wasn't willing to give it up when he was first diagnosed with PD.

He slotted his desire to play in one corner of his mind and tucked his awareness of multiple physical limitations (sore shoulder, stumbling feet, stooped back, and weak muscles) in another corner of his mind. Our answer: try a training program to see if continuing to play was feasible.

After he finished his extensive physical therapy program, Dean and I practiced hitting balls on a court with no net the next spring at least twice a week. At home, he took the initiative of exercising on the floor with the program that he received from his clinic physical therapist. He jogged in place at the kitchen sink. After his naps, he regularly stretched all his leg and arm muscles to fight off the rigidity.

His hard work paid off. He was able to play fairly competitive tennis with his buddies the entire 2006 indoor tennis season! He felt victorious. I thought he deserved a Gold Medal.

As the disease continued to work on his agility and stamina, his buddies and I adjusted his playing time for the 2007 year. He would warm up and play for approximately 30 minutes. I would finish out the hour and a half session. The third year, he could only warm up for 10 minutes before I took over. In his mind, as long as he was on the court hitting balls, he was playing tennis.

He knew that he might fall again. I feared that he might fall again. Our message is not to be unsafe on a tennis court. The message is to stay passionately involved in something you love to do, even when it takes enormous work to do it. In an effort to be honest about the disease, it was a spiral of adjustments for my husband. He eventually had to give up playing tennis because his balance was too precarious. After he no longer could play, he became an enthusiastic fan. His tennis group continued to include him in pizza parties at the end of every season. He enjoyed watching them and sharing in the post-match discussion over the pizza. Their support was of tremendous benefit to his self esteem.

The adventure attitude is having the belief that you can make the impossible happen, but not becoming devastated when it doesn't.

An Optimistic Attitude

Pessimism is easy, optimism takes work. It may sound trite to recommend staying positive when one finds himself hurled into a fiercely raging storm, but it's absolutely true. Lewy Body Dementia can be a nasty disease. With positive thinking, there is a greater chance that the inevitable anger, rage, and frustrations will be manageable. Manageable means better care — less pain and discomfort. With less pain and discomfort, the patient should be able to continue doing more things independently. The more he can do, the less the caregiver must do. It is a win-win situation.

An "I-Can" Attitude

Instilling a belief inside a person that he can continue doing difficult tasks will help maintain an optimistic attitude. If Dean was to stay motivated, I had to adjust his environment to allow him to use his strengths and get around his weaknesses. Before being diagnosed, Dean retired and I went back to work. He assumed the duties of a house husband. When his memory started to fail him, he began to have trouble doing his jobs around the house. We talked about the problems he was having, and made some simple adjustments to allow him to continue housekeeping successfully.

I circled the start buttons on the dishwasher, labeled the stove burner knobs, and painted an arrow on the clothes dryer controls to help him visually see how to operate the appliances. I painted a big H and C on the shower dial that he could see without his glasses.

A big digital kitchen clock listing the day of the week, time and date helped him keep track of his days. He maintained a calendar of activities and wrote down all grocery needs on a pad by the calendar. He used his pocket notebooks to jot down ideas and reminders to stay on top of daily tasks. Misplacing personal items such as glasses, wallet, money and keys was a real downer. He worked very hard to put these items back immediately in one of two bureau top baskets. When out of the house, I carried his wallet in my pocket or purse until we both started wearing fanny packs.

It was easier to assume an I-Can attitude inside the house than out in public. Our message is to brave it. I took Dean everywhere. When he needed a wheelchair for long distances, I had a hitch put on our car. A bicycle rack worked beautifully as a wheelchair mount to hold his wheelchair and my bike. He was able to continue going to picnics, the Aquarium, and outdoor concerts: all things he loved to do with our granddaughters.

The "I-Can" attitude can be severely challenged when trying to master the use of public restrooms. If we had not developed a good sense of humor at our mishaps, we might have given up our master plan to live life as an adventure. On one occasion, when Dean was still walking by himself, he went into the men's room at a highway rest stop. It was before he stopped wearing belts. He was gone well over 30 minutes, and I was becoming worried about him. He finally came out with a quick shuffle holding his pants up with both hands. He hustled into the car and said "GO!" We left a little attendant man shuffling toward the car carrying Dean's skivvies. Apparently, Dean couldn't get the belt undone in time. He had all he could do, to get his feet out of the trouser legs, once he was able to sit. He got the wet underwear off and managed to get his pants back on, but the effort nearly exhausted him. He left the belt and the under shorts on the floor for fear of falling if he bent over to pick them up. But he almost got caught! The elder attendant was shuffling after him with the incriminating skivvies waving in the breeze.

We found that if we wanted to continue having fun outside the house, we needed to continue to tweak the bathroom routine. After the highway rest stop disaster, Dean wore no belts and switched to elastic-waisted pants. When he began to have balance issues, we searched for the family restrooms that I could enter with him. If we were with a male friend who felt comfortable helping Dean, they would use the men's room together. As a last resort, I asked someone to stand guard while I went into the men's room. On one occasion, I had to take Dean into the handicapped stall of the ladies room. He accepted these modifications because he felt it was worth it. We felt we had to step out in faith and make the most of what we had.

Caregivers Need an I-Can Attitude.

It is also extremely important for the caregiver to believe in herself. Most people get hurled into a caregiving role without much warning. Making life decisions for another person is scary. As a professional, I was trained to handle all aspects of a disease; and yet, it was more than I felt I could do at times. I took my inspiration from Dean. As he inched forward striving to overcome, I would dig deep to find solutions to make his journey easier. It was a day-to-day decision. I would wake up in the morning and say to myself, "Here we go again." I believe we are all capable of more than we initially think we can do.

An Attitude of Gratitude

As I took the time to thank others for their kindnesses, I realized how fortunate we were to have so many people fighting the battle with us. Expressing my gratitude actually helped me maintain my optimism. Having received was the best way for me to learn to be compassionate to others, especially toward Dean.

The Attitude of Compassion

Our days were not all fun and games. The day that Dean tripped on a crack in the sidewalk on our neighborhood walk, my emotions shot from anger at him and myself, embarrassment that I hadn't prevented the fall, disappointment, rage at the disease, and panic. It was easy to get him up from the floor in the house where I could put something in front of him. I had nothing but open space on our walk. Fortunately, the lady who lived near by saw us and came to our aid. I had not met her before, but could clearly see that she possessed an I-Can attitude toward life. She was probably in her seventies, working in her yard, wearing fashion jeans and wedge shoes with 3 inch heels. When she asked if she could help, I answered that I wasn't sure because Dean was fairly heavy. Her reply was, "I may not look it, but I'm pretty strong. Let's give it a try." Dean wasn't hurt. With each of us helping, he popped right up, and we went on our way. She was, surely, the right person at the right moment on that day. Her compassionate help bolstered both of our spirits.

Compassion, the expression of understanding, is the result of empathy. Not everyone has the capacity to empathize. We were always deeply moved by the many simple acts of compassion that we received. Amazingly, when someone took the time to reach out to us, we seemed to make more of an effort to reach out to each other. It enabled me to deal with Dean's helplessness with a bit more patience and devotion. He, in turn, responded to all my efforts with deep-felt appreciation.

Tender touch can be a very powerful way to express compassion. It kept the closeness, the humanness, the intimacy of our relationship alive. I always held his arm or hand when walking, but that was on a need-to-do basis. The choice to sit together on our two person sofa for some snuggle time was a balm for our broken hearts. He needed to feel that he was still cherished in his broken state. I needed to feel the strength of his arm around my shoulder. In those few moments I was not a caregiver, but the wife of a loving husband.

I doubt if all the people who reached out to us realized that their efforts were more than sustaining. We actually found that we began doing nice things for other people that we saw on the ragged edge. The tenderness and compassion that we received was paid forward.

Compassionate gestures are so powerful that I will end this chapter briefly describing several types of kindnesses. Dean and I had to learn to accept these kind acts. Had we not let others into our world, we wouldn't have experienced the gratitude that helped us stay positive.

The Giving of Time

Family and friends volunteered to relieve me. Some came for a few hours so I could shop or play tennis. Others actually spent overnights with Dean during the periods when his care was fairly extensive.

My son took care of Dean for four days when I presented information at a therapy conference. Since my son did not have a shower bench and Dean could be shaky on his feet, I told Todd not to let him take a shower while I was gone. He did anyway. When he realized how slippery Dean was wet, my 6'-3" son just took off his shoes and got into the shower with his dad to be sure Dean didn't fall. That was truly getting into the trenches. Once they were both dry and safe, it was worthy of a good laugh.

The Gift of Thoughtfulness

One neighbor came in to talk politics with Dean while his wife hit tennis balls with me. Both gave to us just what we each needed: firing him up and calming me down. One group brought us a whole party. They provided everything for a picnic. We merely had to eat and laugh. Getting emails from a 10- year-old nephew asking me to give Uncle Dean a hug did not take much time, but those few minutes gave me an allusion of normalcy, and a quiet awareness that out there somewhere, someone cared.

The Gift of Family

My brother provided the painful therapy to get Dean's shoulders working again. My sister-in-law and her sister completely cleaned my house one weekend. The beauty they created stayed with me for weeks. Our daughter sat at her dad's knee and talked, or took him out for ice cream. My son listened as I ranted about all my fears, concerns, and gripes. Our daughter-in-law and son-in-law supported as they were able. Everyone contributed according to their talents.

No one helped us feel the sense of true compassion better than our two little granddaughters. They spent overnights with us throughout all phases of Dean's illness. When he could go on walks, albeit walking slowly, our granddaughters would hold Dean's hands to be sure he didn't walk alone. When he needed a wheelchair for our walks, they held onto the wheelchair. They jumped in bed with him in the mornings. They shared special snacks with him. They blew him kisses with enthusiasm.

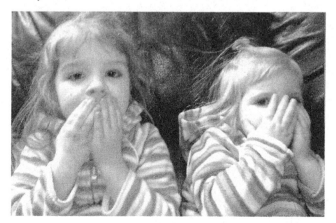

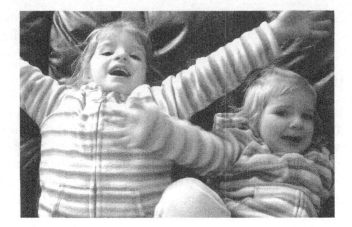

His physical decline with messy spills and abnormal movements was never an issue with them; he was just Grampa. In them, we saw true unconditional love and acceptance. The joy they created for us is immeasurable.

Chapter 4

Taking Control by Scheduling
in the Fun Things

There's an opportune time to do things, a right
time for everything on the earth:
—Ecclesiastes 3 The Message

I am not an obsessive optimist, trying to paint a pretty picture of an ugly situation. The reality that Dean and I were fighting a battle for his survival was squarely in my face. My future was crumbling. We both felt like victims. Of the two of us, I felt more like the victim than he did. I had to fight daily, even hourly on some days, to soak in his touch, his warmth, his smile, and his funny comments. All would help me avoid being angry and feeling sorry for myself. The worst time of the day was 11:00 p.m. to 1:00 a.m. I couldn't bury my feelings of hopelessness in care activities at the end of the day. I was alone with the fears, the unknowns, the remorse, and the anger circling my mind in an incessant loop of thoughts. I could be completely exhausted, but not able to shut my mind off to get needed sleep.

Unfortunately, the more I wallowed in my negative thoughts, the more impatient I would become with Dean. It became a vicious cycle. As I felt sorry for myself, the worse I was in my caregiving. This produced more guilt, which brought me to an even lower level of sadness. When I would think rationally, I realized that the situation imposed on me was not Dean's fault, anymore than contracting the disease was his fault.

Dean was a very kind and gentle man to all who knew him. He could have ranted and complained as each new liberty was stripped from his day. But he didn't. He continued to focus on the positives in his life. He taught me that we had to make the joy happen. Without the decisions to do things that brought fun memories, humor, and belly laughs; we would both become victims: me to my own sad mind-set and him to my poor caregiving. We purposefully created the memories and the moments.

a time to weep and a time to laugh;
—Ecclesiastes 3:4 RSV

Purposely Add Humor

Dean's use of humor was priceless. It was the glue that held us together. Because we chose to laugh at ourselves, we built a treasure trove of great memories. Funny experiences happened every day, when I began to look for them. A funny comment could get me through the day, a belly laugh held me together for a week.

Dean was good at one-liner comments. He could twist a typical, daily situation into a humorous scenario. After his walking became unsteady, I needed to routinely trail slightly behind him with my hand holding his safety belt anytime he walked in the house. On one walk from the bedroom to the kitchen, he said, "How do you like always being relegated to the end of the parade?" Thereafter, I found myself smiling when we 'paraded' through our house several times a day.

Neither of us had ever been in a situation like this before. The screw-ups could be very funny, and we made the most of the clumsiness in my care techniques. On several occasions, as I was washing his back, I nipped him with the sharp edge of my engagement ring. He teasingly yelped, "If you don't quit wounding me with that thing, I will be sorry that I ever bought it for you." I would then routinely smile as I guarded him from my ring.

Dean had the ability to state an absurdity with a straight face to lighten up my intensity. I really struggled with his slowness. He was not an impetuous person before he was sick; but he could be a sloth when doing daily activities after the disease kicked in. I tried not to nag at him to hurry up, but I was very good at nagging. It was a difficult habit to break. To help speed up morning care, Dean elected to have a buzzed haircut for the few hairs he still had on the top of his head. One morning as we were beginning the shave and shower routine, he stopped before getting into the shower to COMB his hair. I blurted out with ragged impatience, "Now, what are you doing?" Without hesitation, he said, "Checking for snarls!" He smiled, and we both cracked up.

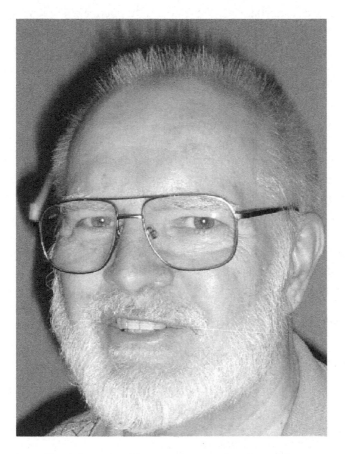

Once I realized how good spontaneous laughter felt, I purposefully added humorous activities to our days. We rarely traveled without listening to a radio station that played comedy 24 hours a day. I picked movies that were comedies, and read him funny emails and hilariously funny books. Our reading time after breakfast was a prized time of the day for both of us.

If you can't make it better, you can laugh at it.
Erma Bombeck

Scheduling Weekly Activities

Dean and I not only needed to laugh, we needed to DO activities. To schedule and plan excursions was no longer a simple task. The more unstable mentally and physically that he became, the more demanding the planning became. These activities may be more laborious than some families can do. My intent is to show that vacations can still happen, even when a spouse is in a wheelchair. The importance of all the outings and purposefully scheduled fun activities was to keep Dean looking to the future and to keep me focused on the positives. This section will offer suggestions that caregivers might do to maintain a sense of fun in each day.

Dean and I planned activities for every day of the week. It kept him looking toward tomorrow. It could be something as simple as grocery shopping, which we did together every Wednesday for a long time. We used an electric scooter after his stamina decreased. Unfortunately, I had to take his scooter license away when people kept getting in his way in the grocery aisles.

We attended church functions, especially those that included food. Twice a week, we played games or shuffleboard at the Senior Center. In the evenings, we went to the music concerts or enjoyed pot luck suppers at the Center. Most of these activities were free. Dean worked hard to remember what day it was, and what activity he needed to be prepared to do.

Scheduling Big Vacations

We took three cruises during our LBD adventure. For two of the three, we had overnight flights to Europe to start the cruise. Dean planned, exercised, and read in preparation for these vacations. All trips required more than simple preparations from me. Unlike all the other vacations during our married years, he could do nothing to help me. After I purchased cancellation insurance, I prayed.

For the last cruise in May 2009 I needed a boatload of prayer. He had been walking well and thinking quite clearly in November of 2008 when we booked the cruise. The new medications seemed to be working very well. Four friends were so excited, they agreed to visit Spain and cruise the Mediterranean Sea with us.

In February of 2009 the bottom dropped out of his bucket of health. Dean had to be admitted to the hospital for a violent drug reaction after taking two pills of a drug prescribed by an urologist. It robbed him of all function. Nothing he said made any sense. Some of the words were not even English sounding words. He was submerged into a fantasy world, and nothing I did was able to bring him back. Unfortunately, all the coordination in his legs left as well. When I tried to transfer him from the bed to his wheelchair, both legs flew up into the air as if he was a puppet, and someone had pulled the strings. I was able to direct him into the chair before he crashed to the floor, but it was not easy.

When he came back home after the three day stay, he was not significantly better. I felt the trip to Spain slipping away. It took over a week for him to begin to stand, transfer and do short walks to the bathroom without total exhaustion.

In March, I was ready to call and cancel the trip, but Dean begged me not to give up. Few people believed that he would be able to endure a trip as extensive as flying across the Atlantic Ocean for 10 hours. I didn't believe he would be able to do it. I was scared beyond words to even consider a trip that demanding.

He never lost his belief that we would be able to go to Spain with dear friends. As long as he was willing to work toward that goal, I was willing to work with him. He walked almost every day for six weeks. We started out slowly walking in the house. When his stamina improved, we ventured out for neighborhood walks with a rolling walker that had a seat. On those first walks I needed to put a chair on the sidewalk by our porch before we left. He would be sweating profusely and utterly exhausted when we returned to the house. At that point, I had to live on his optimism.

In reality, he made the trip and loved it. It turned out to be a wonderful vacation for all six of us.

More Information About Vacations

Vacations were essential for both of us. Long outings remained a big focus. We planned small and large trips about every three months. Early in the disease process, we flew to various scenic cities. Later, we chose cities within driving range and stayed in condominiums or hotel rooms that I could set up similarly to his home environment. There were places that we had long planned to see together. We managed to see most of them.

There are many advantages to traveling and sight seeing with someone in a wheelchair. Parking in the handicapped area was closer, fees were reduced, and people were especially accommodating. When we went to Walt Disney World in Florida, we rented an electric scooter. It was wonderful for him to be self-propelled and not Judy-propelled.

Tips on Flying

Early in our travels, we missed our connecting flight out of New York because of long lines through Customs. This bad experience taught me to always arrange wheelchair assistance from the airline representatives. The wheelchair attendants were experienced at getting us to the next gate the shortest possible way and helping us get through Customs. I didn't have to worry about my husband; I only had to manage the carry-on articles. In Atlanta, special-needs check-out terminals were a tremendous benefit.

Packing traveling items in a carry on bag helped make the flights tolerable. Blow up neck collars provided some head support for sleeping comfortably in the plane or car. Sleep masks blocked the light. Raisins, nuts, gum and snacks sustained us between meals.

Dean was always able to walk on his own for short distances when we flew, but I was concerned that he might lose his balance if the plane ride became bumpy from turbulence. I reserved seats as close to a lavatory as possible.

Certainly traveling with other people eased the stresses for me. On one trip when we were alone, I used a limo service to pick us up at the airport. It provided a second set of hands to load Dean and his chair when we were both very tired after a long flight.

Consider cancellation insurance. We did and actually had to use it once. It was a small price to pay to keep him motivated to work hard and stay focused on the next big trip.

Tips for Car Trips

When Dean stopped driving, I traded in both cars and bought one that would allow Dean to stretch out as much as possible. We ended up with a small SUV that almost completely reclined the front seat. With an extra chaise lounge cushion on his seat, he was fairly comfortable for a two hour window of time between restroom breaks. He also used the neck collar and two other pillows for his arms.

We learned to be prepared with a bag containing bottles of water, snacks, cell phone and charger, GPS, maps, and a travel folder containing all the particulars of the trip. A separate bag was filled with an emergency urinal and extra clothes. Since I had to do all the driving, we both stayed focused by listening to audio books that I checked out at the library.

When we got to our destination, I set up the bedroom just as I had Dean's particulars set up at home. This worked for a cruise, condo, friend's home, or motel. We worked around his nap times and had great memory-making vacations. I made sure I didn't have anything to do on the calendar for at least three days after we got home.

When Dean needed to use a wheelchair almost all of the time, I had a hitch mounted to the car by a specialist recommended by the salesman at the dealership. We bought a bicycle rack that would hold his wheelchair and my bike. This system worked well for us, but might be difficult for people who are not strong enough to mount the wheelchair onto the rack. Most car trunks are big enough to store a folded wheelchair. Of course, all of this discussion assumes that the caregiver is able to transfer the spouse in and out of the car safely.

Scheduling Fun When Staying Around Home

Family Reunions

Family get-togethers can be memory makers. We had three in five years. Relatives came from all over the country for a " Visit with Dean" party. I set out scrapbooks of ancestors and made a genealogy tree with all the family members attached to their particular branches. Cousins who had never met had fun seeing where they were connected. We placed copies of old pictures on a table for sharing. Dean and his first cousins were more than willing to tell family stories to the younger generations.

Local Activities

Afternoon excursions allowed us to get out of the house for a few hours and required very little effort on Dean's part. We used unique events: birthday parties, short trips to visit old friends, movies, or visits with grandkids for our excursions. Mid afternoon was a good time to go to movies at the dollar saver theaters. They were not crowded, and we could always get a seat that gave Dean more leg room.

Eating out was always a pleasant activity. I got a break from cooking. Dean got a variety of food and a chance to visit with other people. We regularly attended church potlucks, met friends in restaurants, or ate pizza at Concerts in the Park. It might be important for other caregivers to realize that Dean was willing to do almost any social event if I was with him. He could become very anxious if he was left with other people for very long. Amazingly, he would be at his best, both physically and mentally, when we were visiting with others.

Unique Events

TV sports specials were unique events. During the NCAA basketball tournament every year, we each filled out a bracket and competed with other family members. Did I want to watch basketball continuously for three weekends? A resounding "No"; but Dean did. With the motivation of the bracket picks, each game became important to him.

We enjoyed Breakfast at Wimbledon for tennis and the Super Bowl for football. It was all part of putting invigorating events on the calendar and into Dean's life.

At-Home Leisure Fun

We made the most of Dean's strengths and supported his weaknesses to keep his home activities fun. Games playing needed a progression of adjustments throughout the course of the disease. It can stay fun until it obviously causes frustration. We teamed up to play board games and do crossword puzzles — both of us trying to answer the same questions. Our goal was spending fun time together. It didn't matter if anybody won. I needed to keep score for both of us for most games.

Dean had the most stamina for games when we played with other people. Even our grandchildren could keep him thinking creatively. He enjoyed their kiddy games. All he had to do was roll the dice, move a game piece ahead, and laugh

Interactive games on the television should be tried before purchasing. Some of the games require less quick movements than others. Trial and error will determine which are appropriate. Senior centers might be a good place to try games before purchasing them.

Start a New Hobby or Resurrect an Old One

We gave the old high school coronet a try. At first he could only work the keys for about 3-5 minutes. With practice several times a week, he built up both the stamina in his arms and lips to play for 20 minutes. He and I needed to appreciate the big picture. He was playing for fun not creating beautiful music. He loved playing again, and his finger strength and breath control increased. Some days he enjoyed sitting in the family room whistling his old tunes. Any form of making music works both the brain and the muscles.

Caregivers may be able to encourage some new creative craft that will be as effective as playing an instrument. I would not; however, recommend that someone with LBD take up whittling. Reading, painting with water colors, antique collecting may all be examples of hobbies that someone might enjoy doing. An elderly friend of ours lost the ability to play his trumpet because he had extensive arthritis in his hands. He found that he enjoyed making tape recordings of all his old vinyl records. His friends started bringing their records to him by the dozens. He spent several years happily recording hundreds of cassette tapes that his wife listened to in the car for many years.

Reading together was very enjoyable for us. When Dean's vision became blurry, reading was impossible; but, listening to audio books was still fun and kept him solidly awake. I read him one series of frivolous mystery books that made us both belly laugh at the silly situations [18].

Unscheduled Activities and Outright Zany Activities

We cut the tension that surrounded our every minute with the frivolous, the goofy, and the unexpected, spontaneous and sometimes zany activities. I recommend activities similar to these that were spontaneous. The zany could have been disastrous.

Spontaneous

We would get ice cream at 11:00 a.m., if we felt like an ice cream outing. Ice cream runs were never an extravagance. They were essential memory maker moments. I might have to attend ice-cream-eaters anonymous in the future, but during his illness, it was survival food.

We would haul all the breakfast meal out to the deck at 6:30 a.m. to listen to the birds.

We replayed old slide shows of past travels or looked at old scrapbooks.

Some mornings we might leisurely sit at the kitchen table for an hour and think back on old memories or ponder the mysteries of the universe.

Zany

Zany unsafe activities are not recommended.

I was sorely naïve and/or overzealous with my poor dear husband's safety on a few occasions. Thankfully results ended happily. With the intent to inform, enjoy our zany experiences. Of all the many fun days that we shared, it is these zany ones that I remember the most vividly.

- We purchased two bicycles during the early phase of the disease. After a half hour drive, we had to return them for a refund – Dean had fallen when he tried to turn a corner.

- We rented a three-wheeled bike for him at a state park and ventured out on a bike path. This path, unbeknownst to me, had a 'ferocious' hill. I pushed my bike against his trike and got both bikes up the hill. To my dismay, there was a big down slope on the other side! I will never forget the image of Dean cresting the hill and gaining momentum as he sped downward on the path. And I will ever be grateful that something inspired that little old lady to move off the path just before Dean came careening by on his three-wheeled-trike. I am sure his cycle had brakes. He just couldn't find them. That was definitely an ice cream day.

- The worst decision and zaniest outing I ever organized was a trip to an Omni Max theater midway into the disease process. Dean was still walking independently without support, but was somewhat shaky on uneven ground. The ushers "ushered" us to a high row of seats and "ordered" us into the middle of the aisle. At that early stage, I wasn't assured of my caregiver responsibilities. I should have refused the inside seats and insisted on an aisle seat, but I caved in and let them march us into the very center of the row. Dean made it into the row easily. He wasn't tired going IN. After the show, it dawned on me just how very narrow and steep the seat rows were. It felt like I was asking him to walk sideways 25 feet on the edge of the Grand Canyon. I held onto him for dear life, and had horrific visions of him catching a toe and rolling over hundreds of people on the way to the bottom of the theater. After that day, I did not let anyone tell him what to do. I learned to say, "No", if any situation did not fit his needs.

Persevere in Your Efforts To Add Fun To Each Day

It is easy to give up without big ideas that take some work. But don't. I've offered you some ideas about managing this disease adventure with a fun attitude, but it takes work to make your ideas come alive. It takes work that you and the person in your care must be willing to do together. Your scheduled fun will probably be much different than what Dean and

I enjoyed doing. Certainly all decisions should be based on medical status and limitations. The important thing is to seek out activities that add zest to the day.

I always had a vacation looming in the future to keep my sanity. Mostly, I was trying to encourage Dean to keep moving. Yes, we pushed to the limit at every stage; recovered our nerves, and then, rejoiced in a captured memory. We found many 'carrots' that inspired both of us to get out of bed each morning and make the decision to celebrate life.

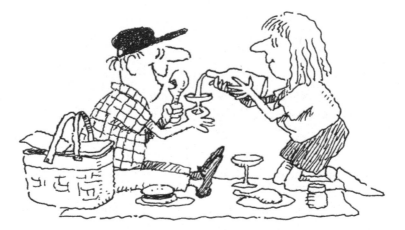

Chapter 5

Talking about Burn-out

A right time to hold on and another to let go,
—Ecclesiastes 3: The Message, The Wisdom Books

Caregivers can get to a point, when one more minute of giving, is too much. Nothing of the self is left except a charred frame. This is burn-out, the ultimate negative reaction for the caregiver. At that moment, if she "can't make changes, she needs to make changes". Specifically, if she can't change things in ways that promote peace of mind while providing care, she needs to remove herself from the caregiving role. And conversely, if there is no other option for the care of the loved one, she needs to make changes in how she is providing care.

This is critically important for both persons. Elder abuse has become a big issue. The victim of a disease should not become the victim of an overwrought caregiver. From the caregiver's perspective, self sacrifice to the point of ill health serves nobody.

There may come a time when caring for a person in the home is too dangerous. That can certainly be true if the person is having violent hallucinations and fears for his/her life. Strong medications may be needed that will require a hospitalization for medical management. It can also prove too dangerous to care for someone at home when physical skills are very deficient. People that can't stand while living in a nursing facility are lifted out of bed with a mechanical hydraulic lift to be sure that the caregivers and the person do not experience injury during transfers.

On the other hand, if a person can remain in his home surrounded by loving, caring people, his quality of life may well be superior to being in a facility. A balance is needed. While caring for another person, it's absolutely imperative that caregivers make time for themselves.

I speak from my own experience. As Dean's mind and body deteriorated, my time commitment seemed to be 36 hours instead of 24.[19] In the late stages of the disease, he had many days when he needed constant attention. On occasion, he even called out for me in his sleep. These were the deer-in-the-headlight days for me. I was so overwhelmed that I couldn't do anything to get myself out of danger.

Fortunately, my pastor set me straight. At a counseling session, he ministered to the broken part of me. I was shocked when he told me to start wearing make-up. He told me that both Dean and I needed me to look more upbeat; and he was right. I made many changes after that talk that enabled me to step outside of the chaos.

Making Changes to Care for the Caregiver Physically and Mentally

May these changes that I made trigger possible changes to help other caregivers recharge physically, emotionally, and spiritually.

Find a new look.

Attending a make-up party at the church made me feel like a teen-ager again. A new hair cut and new clothes gave me a fresh look at life. Feeling good on the outside seemed to fill in the gaps I had inside.

Do something physically tiring.

After a year of no tennis, I began playing again. Tennis may not be the game of choice for everyone; but exercise of any kind is a frustration buster. I took walks, rode my bike in the neighborhood, worked in the yard, cleaned out the garage, and stripped wallpaper off the bathroom and hallway walls while Dean took naps.

Carve out personal time.

With the help of paid and volunteer helpers, several small blocks of time were built into my personal schedule. In many communities, a council on aging consultant will come to the home to discuss help services that the community has to offer. More is mentioned about this in Chapter 13. Savoring my specialty coffee during grocery shopping became an hour in Utopia. I was free to be me.

I used volunteer buddies to make my tennis times work. Dean and I made a list of neighborhood buddies whom he would enjoy spending some time with each week. They were each willing to come and sit with him to let me get out and play tennis. For two years, I maintained a schedule of guys one night a week. Dean had a little party with treats, while I was out smashing away my frustrations on the tennis court. Both of us had a fun evening. When we talked later, we each had many new conversational tidbits to share.

Do something that relaxes the mind.

A few games of Solitaire on the computer or email messaging with friends could also serve to relax me after Dean went to bed. Some caregivers enjoy needle crafts or reading. I tended to sleep better if I cleared my mind before going to bed.

Journaling May Provide Spiritual Rejuvenation

My greatest defense against burn-out was my personal letter writing conversations with God. In those God-letters, I could be completely honest with my feelings. Everything came up from the depths and took shape on my paper pages. The process within the letter writing is still amazing to me whenever I reread those pages.

Some people may label journaling just an act of freely writing or a form of meditation. I felt I was making a true connection with a supreme being. The process may be helpful no matter what we label it. What worked for me was finding a way to get my feelings to the surface. When the negatives were out, I could deal with them. When I cleared out the garbage thinking, I seemed to refill with more compassion. This was a good thing, because Dean increasingly needed all the compassion and time that I could give.

Even more important than expressing my feelings, the free-writing produced a sense of peace. That is the power story. Amazing words came through my fingers after I dumped my feelings onto the page. I would stop thinking my thoughts, wait, and then free-write whatever thoughts came into my head. At times, an answer to a perturbing caregiving dilemma would surface. Sometimes, an overflowing of gratitude would come forth for all the good things in my life. Frequently, I would just write, "You are loved", as if my invisible writing partner knew I dearly needed to hear those words.

An example of journaling is presented in **Chapter 16, Spiritual Support**.

Awakening After Burn-Out Passed

I realized that care for the caregiver can make a difference. I moved past my burn-out and found a spiritual revitalization that is hard to describe in words. During the days of extreme pressures with Dean's declining health in the last year, I experienced moments of an amazing phenomenon. These experiences were both emotional and spiritual. When I would allow myself to 'step' out from under the heavy weight of my circumstances, I would find validations that, "Yes, I AM loved," and "I am not alone" in the unexpected, unexplainable events of my day. As humor brought joy, so did the serendipity. The first flowers in March, baby birds in a nest by my door, or rainbows after a shower became personal treasures. It seemed that after I came out of my period of burn-out, I could get high on life. I had moments where I would find myself in a virtual reality scenario with the unexpected events of nature, love, and laughter streaming to me in 3-D.

A song by Josh Groban [20] described these moments of hyper-alertness. The title is *Awake*. He sings that he knows the relationship with his loved one will change; MUST change. He contemplates how he will carry on if he should lose his lover. His song-answer is to stay awake. If he keeps his eyes open wide, he speculates that he will be able to memorize every detail of his love…and everything will indeed, stay the same. For the last six months of Dean's life, my eyes were open wide, taking in all the details. It was…

a time to love,
—Ecclesiastes 3:8 RSV

Chapter 6

Understanding the Physical Changes

Why is Walking Important?

a time to break down and a time to build up;
—Ecclesiastes 3:3 RSV

In neurological degenerative diseases, such as Parkinson disease (PD) and Lewy Body Dementia (LBD), loss of coordination and stamina may be the first indications that something is medically wrong. Stooped posture, shuffling walking steps, and fear of falling may be good reasons to have a doctor and a physical therapist assess any movement disorders.

The main goal is to keep our loved ones moving as safely as possible throughout the course of the disease. It does not have to be a steady downhill loss of skills with LBD. A progression of decline can be expected, but home exercises can make a huge difference in slowing down the decline. Research in 2009 showed that walking could be improved in patients with PD with a rehabilitation program.[21] My experience with my husband tends to assure me that exercise can be very valuable with LBD as well.

Why Work With a Physical Therapist?

Physical therapists are trained to help people with balance issues. After a thorough evaluation, the therapist would set up a rehabilitation program intended to improve strength, coordination, and agility. Patients willing to fully participate in that program should improve walking abilities and experience more energy.

Similar to a car mechanic working on a broken car, a PT is a body mechanic and must first identify all the parts that don't work. My husband was hurting his leg muscles every time he played tennis. The PT found several muscles that were too weak and too tight for healthy tennis motions. Once he was rehabilitated, Dean was able to play tennis for three more years without any leg pains.

Some people, just like cars, become worn out. Many parts don't work. Unfortunately, science is not yet able to replace brain areas that have damage. For a person with a neuromotor disease such as LBD or PD, the best the PT can do is fill up the tank with as much strength and agility as the person can muster. The stronger the muscles are, the longer it will take before loss of abilities is noticeable. Working with a professional should provide an exercise program that is effective without experiencing pain from too strenuous an approach.

All discussion in this book assumes that transfers and walking by the patient will be done in a safe manner for both the patient and the caregiver and approved by the medical team. That stated, it is important to know that PTs have many approaches to teach caregivers how to help their loved ones continue to walk. We teach appropriate use of canes and walkers to promote safety in the home.

It is critically important for families to become informed about safe and unsafe walking patterns. People who are slowly losing gross motor skills may not realize that the way they are moving is precarious. This is especially true for people with dementia. Therapists can teach caregivers why the walking patterns are changing and what adjustments should be made to either improve the gait patterns or move to a safer mode of transportation such as wheelchair use.

Why Is Exercise Important?

Research suggests that strong exercise may protect the brain cells within the areas of the brain affected by PD.[22] In other words, relatively intense exercise interventions may slow down the disease process. The hope is for movement to be normal for a longer period of time. In LBD, the break down of the brain cells is much faster than in PD. It is especially important to exercise regularly and strenuously for as long as possible with a diagnosis of LBD.

Li Fuzhong and others researched the value of Tai Chi exercise for people with PD. They found that a six-month program helped patients improve stability and reduce falls.[23] After 40 years in PT practice, I can attest that those who can maintain walking skills seem to improve health throughout the body. Following are a few of the benefits observed with maintained walking abilities.

Maintaining leg strength and stamina are obvious benefits. People with strength continue to get out of chairs with minimum need for assistance.

Urinary function and bowel action are helped. Constipation and nausea are not uncommon in LBD. The more walking, the easier bowel movements should be. Nausea may stop or decrease significantly if constipation is not a problem.

Strengthening the vital organs is always a good idea. Keep the motors running. Walking improves heart and lung function. Voice projection can increase from a whisper to normal with better lung output and deeper breaths. The immune system that fights infections and colds runs more efficiently with regular walking. Sweating and increased circulation generated by walking helps to clean out the systems of the body that fight germs. Fatigue is an ever present problem with neurological diseases. Walking can actually help someone gain energy to fight fatigue.

For my husband, there was a connection between walking ability and mental clarity. During the times when Dean needed only minimal assistance to walk, we were able to have great conversations. Conversely, when he was mentally sharp, he was also able to move more assuredly. When he woke foggy-brained in the morning with very little mental clarity, I learned that I would need to provide much more assistance when he tried to stand. On those days, I started with the wheelchair and expected a day with many naps.

As a note, this is not the case for many people with Alzheimer's disease. Cognitive abilities may be severely dysfunctional, but walking abilities can continue to be independent.

It was easy to understand why all Dean's doctors encouraged him to keep walking and exercising from very early in the disease. The type of exercise is not as important as finding something that will be done regularly. Dean played tennis and walked. Other people have reported feeling better with cycling or swimming. This is a personal preference. The body doesn't care how it exercises, just that it does. As a former football player, Dean understood the benefits of staying strong. I needed to organize his walking sessions like an exercise coach, but I didn't have to nag like a drill sergeant.

Equally important is the benefit to the caregiver. All effort that our loved ones generate saves time and energy for us. It's much easier to get someone out of bed, onto the toilet, or into a car when the person with compromised health can stand on his feet with some balance and self control. Many caregivers must give up caregiving when they can no longer lift the sick person. In fact, caregivers, both in homes and in nursing homes, have a high incidence of back problems as a result of trying to move someone who is too weak to help themselves.

Can People With LBD Continue to Walk Up And Down Stairs?

Stairs will become challenging. As long as strength remains good and railings are available, stair climbing should be safe. It's best to consult with a PT early in the disease, before it becomes difficult to step up and down curbs. There are correct ways to help a loved one maneuver on stairs. Assisting in an unsafe manner can cause both people to crash.

When I did PT home health, I was amazed at how many patients had steps leading into their houses, but no railings. Having railings installed is such a small task when compared with the pain, cost, and rehabilitation that would be required after a fall that produced a broken hip. Railings for stairs inside the house are a must as well.

Families might be able to find people who can help install railings by asking within their church, contacting Council on Aging nurses, or checking handy man helpers in the community. If your loved one is to remain in the home, any stair issue will need to be addressed. It is certain that there will be days when the LBD will not allow walking safely on stairs.

Some families may have to adjust the environment if stair climbing is no longer possible. When my father-in-law moved in with us after he had a stroke, we hired a contractor to make our first floor living room into a sleeping area and sitting room for him. Several of my home health patients slept in a reclining chair when they no longer could climb stairs to get to a second floor bedroom.

Standing Is Beneficial.

Even when walking is no longer safe, moving with assistance from bed to chair throughout the day is much easier if the patient has the ability to stand and take one step to transfer into a chair. My husband was able to go out into the community throughout all phases of the disease because he was able to stand with only minimal assistance to get into the wheelchair or into the car.

At times, one or both of Dean's shoulders were very sore; and our sit-to-stand techniques had to accommodate for that pain. He had the least amount of discomfort if he could push to the edge of the chair as much as he could by himself. Then, I needed to provide support as he pushed himself out of the chair to an upright position. I was looking for as much effort from my husband as I could get. One phrase that I frequently used to get him to standing was, "Lean forward to get your nose over your toes". We also used a 1-2-3 counting, rocking system to be sure we were both working together to get him over his feet.

The alternative to a safe stand up transfer is being moved via a pneumatic lift. This is a wonderful piece of equipment to allow a small person to transfer someone who no longer can stand safely. It works well in homes with adequate space. It does not work well to transfer a person into a car. If the goal is to be able to get out of the house to do activities in the community, the caregiver and patient need to work diligently with professionals on safe stand up transferring abilities.

One of our most important safety tips involves protecting the arms. If the caregiver must pull on her spouse to get him upright, a gait belt around the waist is the safest place to apply pressure. Pulling on arms to help someone stand is never a good idea. Bruising of the skin and injury to joints is very likely if a helper pulls on the arms. It is much better for the person, to push himself up and out, or for him to pull against a solid object such as a bar or Super Pole. When he pulls, he activates all the muscles around a joint, protecting that joint from injury. Pulling on a walker to stand up is unsafe and may cause a fall.

Consultations with the physical therapists will help determine when walking and transfers are no longer safe to do. PT's will also be able to recommend and order pertinent equipment.

What Walking Patterns Are Normal or Abnormal?

In early evaluations, doctors will begin looking at walking patterns, noting those that are normal and those that are abnormal. This evaluation process will likely continue throughout the course of the disease.

Normal

People should walk erect, with eyes forward, head level, shoulders back, and hips and knees straight when the foot is in contact with the ground. The arms should swing easily as the feet are moving forward. Footprints in the sand should show how the feet wag from side to side with one foot significantly out in front of the other. Ideally, toes point straight ahead, but many people walk normally with toes rotating outward or inward slightly. People who walk normally can change direction easily without losing their balance. They can start and stop easily as well as walk rapidly or slowly by choice. Normal walking abilities allow anyone to do other tasks while walking such as talking, or carrying packages.

Some environmental situations can affect people with normal balance. Anyone may experience balance issues when walking in the grass or on rough ground. Throw rugs in the home can also create an uneven surface, and should be eliminated where possible. Dean did a big fall in our kitchen before he was diagnosed, when he was walking on the linoleum in stocking feet. Very slippery!

Abnormal Walking in the Early Phase of LBD

In addition to the loss of balance, strength, and coordination; vision changes may affect how someone will walk. It's important to remember that the world of an afflicted person is not the same as our normal world. They walk in strange ways because those ways feel safer to them. If they could walk more normally, they surely would. Following are several different types of walking patterns that might be seen during the progression of the disease.

Shuffling Gait is an early stage, walking pattern most often associated with PD and LBD. The shuffler leans forward all of the time. His head is bent forward so that his eyes look at the ground. He has forward shoulders, a bend at the hips and often a constant bend in the knees. The feet move as if they are in sloppy slippers dragging on the ground. In some people, this pattern of walking is constant and no verbal instructions to pick up the feet will have any effect. This shuffling pattern may be quite safe initially; but at some point in the spiral of decline, special equipment will become necessary to prevent falls.

If I asked my husband to "take BIG steps", he was able to take longer steps and clear his foot for a short while. I used instructions, such as focusing his eyes 20 feet in front of him, when we took our exercise walks in the neighborhood. I didn't nag him about his feet all of the time. For most of Dean's years with the disease, the more walking he did, the more normal his pattern became. Walking was the exercise that helped walking.

Snowballing is a term used to describe an abnormal walking pattern similar to a snowball rolling down a hill. Medical doctors list this abnormality as "festination". It describes the tendency to lean too far forward when walking. As the pace quickens, the feet need to keep moving faster to stay under the body. Eventually, a fall happens. Caregivers can prevent this if they help the person slow down, stop, or stand more upright as soon as snowballing begins. Telling our loved ones to stop won't work. The momentum, once started, will take help to stop. The caregiver will need to intervene immediately before too much speed is generated. Stopping is the best strategy. It's especially important to prevent momentum on a downhill, but anyone can begin to snowball on any surface. The forward posture sets the pattern into motion

When Dean would start to increase his pace, I might be able to get him to slow down, if I asked him to lift his head. More often, I needed to restrain his walker to slow him down. We would stop, take a deep breath, and then resume our walk. Newer walkers with "reverse brakes" like the U-step walker can be helpful in these situations as well.

Abnormal Walking Patterns in Later Phases of LBD

Balance reactions are those automatic movements that someone does to adjust to the force of gravity. Those movements prevent the body from falling to the ground. This is important for caregivers to understand because the LBD destroys these automatic movements. People with normal balance reactions can move their feet outward from the center of the body to prop themselves up, if they feel themselves leaning too far to one side. Healthy people can take a step backward to correct their balance. When the disease stops the ability to correct the balance, the person with PD or LBD will have as much stability as a pencil standing on end.

Caregivers watching for changes in balance skills should observe how much their loved ones swing the arms when walking. If the arms are rigidly held next to the body, the legs will also have a difficult time moving outward to assist balance reactions. All walking will need to be assisted at this stage.

Freezing might be described as trying hard to move the feet, but no forward movement happens. It is often seen after standing, when trying to get started in a forward direction. It may take 15 seconds to get enough shifting in the body to start moving the first foot forward. A caregiver can help decrease freezing by gently encouraging the loved one to reach for an object in front of them, such as the caregiver's hand, a rail, or a piece of furniture. If a walker is the assisting equipment in use, it may help to gently ease the walker forward a few inches, to get the person to begin weight shifting and step forward.

I helped Dean avoid freezing by giving him a visual cue. When I taped red duct tape in front of his chair, he had a visual path for his feet to follow. It also worked well in a line in front of the commode. He realized he needed to continue stepping backward until he had his feet on the red tape. Then, he could reach back to sit down safely.

Stutter Stepping is similar to freezing. When attempting to walk after standing, the feet may move up and down in the same place, without moving forward. If the caregiver can encourage the person to reach forward toward an object, the forward motion might begin. Sometimes I would gently move Dean's walker slightly away from him. As he leaned toward the walker, his feet would step forward. This works best when people are having difficulty understanding verbal directions. If no language problems are evident, the caregiver may get her spouse to take a normal step by telling him to take a big step.

Stutter stepping may initially be observed when someone moves into a darkened area or into a crowded space. The stutter stepping also seems to occur when the person is tired, or maneuvering a turn. These later stage walking patterns are important for caregivers to understand. They indicate that balance is severely affected, and falls could happen. Many people choose to use wheelchairs all the time rather than chance falling at this stage.

Visual Disturbances Can Affect Walking Safety.

My husband would not be able to figure out the flower designs in the carpet. He occasionally would lift his feet very high to be sure he cleared a flower pattern in the rug. On other days, he might not lift high enough to clear the lip of the shower and would bump his toes. Avoiding objects with a sideways movement was very difficult. If I didn't watch his toes and gently guide him sideways, he would have banged his toes on the legs of chairs or furniture every time he walked.

Later in the disease, he thought he saw black cats (hallucinations) in our house and would jerk to get out of the way of a 'nothing'. If I wasn't holding him during those times, he would have been down on the floor. When his vision further failed him in the advanced stage of the disease, he would approach a sofa to sit down and start to sit before turning his back side to the sofa. I would have to talk and 'walk' him through the motions with my hand guidance to get him squared up to sit down safely. These are situations that make standing and walking very unsafe. All should be discussed with the professionals.

Unique Standing Problems to Report to the Doctor

These strange mannerisms may be part of the disease progression or related to a prescription problem. I suggest telling the doctor about all of them.

Buckling in the Knees

The knees just give out when standing and your loved one can sink to the floor. Dean experienced this one entire day and part of one week. After that, it happened infrequently. We never figured out why it happened and never had a solution. It is scary. We called it dropsie in the knees.

Light headedness, dizziness and fainting should be reported to the medical team.

The cause is important to determine. Is blood pressure stable or is it dropping significantly when a person stands? This is called orthostatic hypotension. To rule this out, the blood pressure will need to be taken twice: lying down and then standing.

Are any medications affecting the blood pressure? Is there a medication to help stabilize the blood pressure? Is dehydration a problem? Do compression stockings help? When I asked our pharmacist for suggestions, she reported that adding salt and caffeine to the diet can help elevate the blood pressure. Our doctor concurred. We didn't completely get rid of this until Dean came off one of the memory enhancing drugs.

Decreased sensation in the feet can make walking more difficult.

In the later stages of the disease, Dean lost some feeling in his feet. Rubber soled moccasins gave him the best feel for the ground and also good gripping on linoleum.

With any of these mannerisms, the safest option will be use of a wheelchair. It is a sound suggestion to have a ramp built to allow easy access in and out of the house before the day comes when the spouse can no longer do steps. Maneuvering a wheelchair either up or down even one step is very challenging and can be dangerous. I almost could not get Dean into the house one evening. The next day, I called our Pastor to ask for assistance. A carpenter in our church built us the most beautiful ramp in the neighborhood the next week. It served us well for many years.

Ambulation Equipment

Canes and walkers are valuable for assistance when gait is unstable, especially outside of the house. These tools are best prescribed by a therapist. In the middle stage, Dean did not need an assistive device in the house, but the cane gave him more support on long outings. Our cane had a triangular rubber pad that allowed the cane to stand upright when not being held. Dean kept the cane that he used for outings next to the door with his fanny pack. These items were easy to grab on the way out the door.

As Dean progressively needed more support, we tried various types of walkers with and without wheels or seats. During the later stage, he preferred to push his wheelchair around the house. He was tall and the handles of the wheelchair fit his height the best. He seemed to stand more upright with the wheelchair than the other equipment. I would decide on days when he was less stable that he should sit rather than push. When he was more unstable, he would lean too heavily on the empty wheelchair and it would tip downward, taking him with it. I don't recommend that patients push an empty wheelchair, but some will insist because they feel it is easier. If that is the case, being aware of the tipping is important information.

A gait belt is a must-have tool when walking with a person in the later stages of LBD. It is a sturdy woven belt that can be purchased from a medical supply store. A gait belt is safer than holding on to clothing when assisting with walking. It is safer than holding on to someone's arm. Bruising can occur easily when holding an arm. My husband encouraged me to tell all wives that holding someone up by the pants creates a very uncomfortable "wedgey".

Use of Restraints

There is a movement within the geriatric nursing community to minimize the use of restraints as much as possible in long term care facilities. Even in the hospice facility, nurses were not allowed to have both rails of the bed up because it would be considered a restraint.

The no-restraint policy may not be a good plan when only one caregiver is in a home setting. Most of the time, I used gates on stairs and arranged furniture for safe wandering. I did use a soft restraint around Dean's middle to tie him into the wheelchair on days when he was very confused and very unstable; and I needed five minutes of uninterrupted time. Medical aid stores will be able to explain the pros and cons of various restraints.

To keep Dean in bed at night, I gerry-rigged my own contraption. It worked well for us. A visiting nurse might have excellent suggestions as well.

We purchased a rail that anchored under the mattress for the head side of the bed. After I had Dean all tucked in for the night, I placed the wheelchair at the bottom side of the bed. The wheelchair worked as a fairly good restraint by itself. It was even more effective after I squeezed a long body pillow between the rail and the wheelchair. With the pillow in place, his legs wouldn't bang into the side of the wheelchair. This was a definite improvement. As a failsafe, I hung cow bells on the wheelchair. When it was all set up, it kept him safely in bed or alerted me quickly that he was trying to wander in the middle of the night.

A hospital bed may be the best option for some families. It will have side rails and can be raised or lowered easily for bed care needs. It can be especially helpful if a loved one always lies on the back and no longer is able to maneuver in bed. I would have had to go with a very large bed for Dean. He moved wildly all over the bed throughout the entire disease process. For the month that I used a hospital bed, he was always flailing his arms or legs into the rails of the bed, getting caught or causing bruises.

The importance of this section on restraints is to orient the caregiver to the need for safety when a person is no longer able to make safe decisions. Prevention of a fall is always the best option. A home consultant may be able to offer suggestions that fit your particular restraint needs.

Chapter 7

Helping to Make Self Care Activities Easier

a time to rend, and a time to sew;
—Ecclesiastes 3:7 RSV

All of the items in this chapter will address activities of daily living. These are the many tasks that we don't usually think about until we lose the ability to do them: dressing, bathing, and eating. Parents work very hard during the preschool years to teach children how to be independent in all these areas. After LBD sets in, a person must learn new ways to do these once simple activities if he is to maintain any level of independence.

At times, I found myself thinking that it would be easier to do it myself, than to encourage my husband, Dean, to stay active in his own daily care. But, as with a small child, great pride can be fostered with accomplishment of difficult tasks. For adults, as well as, with small children, tricks and assists can be offered to level the playing field. When zippers are impossible to do, adjustments are a must.

Why Does a Person With LBD Have So Much Trouble Doing the Little Daily Activities?

The mechanism of the disease attacks the fine motor skills of the fingers and the movements of the arms in several ways. The person's coordination progressively declines. In the lower part of the body, this affects balance and coordination needed for safe walking. In this chapter, motor deficits of the hands and arms will be explained.

Weakness

Specific muscle weakness results from disuse, not as deterioration of the muscles specifically. The inability to coordinate movements can look like weakness. Dean would drop the milk carton onto the floor as if it were a bowling ball. I bought small containers of milk, which helped for awhile. When the disease progressed further, I had to pour all his fluids for him. He could manage the cup. During the advanced stage of the disease, he could not control a cup or glass. I gave him all his fluids in toddler cups with lids to prevent having to change his clothes several times a day. The first time he dropped a cup, he burned his leg with hot coffee. On some days, I had to hold the cup to his lips and feed him. With the waxing and waning, these inabilities could change from day-to-day or hour-to-hour.

Tremors, Stiffness, and Rigidity

Coupled with the weakness and in-coordination, stiffness and rigidity in most joints make movements difficult. Watching someone with LBD pick up small items is like watching someone try to tie a bow while wearing cooking mitts. The movements of the fingers become awkward. All joints of the body develop some amount of rigidity coupled with a lack of sensation. This may be easier to understand if you imagine trying to fit a car key into the lock of a car when the fingers inside big mittens are very stiff with cold. Adding to that picture, the fingers inside the mittens keep dropping the keys into a snow pile.

And lastly, the arms lose the ability to swing freely. This can be seen during walking. Arms hang close to the body and no longer swing in tandem with the movements of the feet. The shoulder stiffness makes it difficult to put the hands into the sleeves of clothing the same way as was done in the past.

Using Exercise To Improve Fine Motor Skills

Exercise really can make a difference. Coordination and stiffness can be improved to allow more independence in daily activities. The following examples will help explain the various goals of exercises and the benefit that each type of exercise can provide. Videos may be available from your doctor or an occupational therapist, showing the simple movement exercise routines that can be done daily to keep shoulder and elbow range of motion. Our neurology department offered a day-long seminar. One of the speakers taught an easy-to-do exercise program for the whole body. Working with an occupational therapist on all of these areas can greatly improve self care for the patient.

Learn an Exercise Routine.

Dean lifted 3 pounds 30 times for almost a year at our fitness center after being discharged from the PT clinic. He also stretched his arms upward, sideways and backward with elbows as straight as possible.

Dean worked his arms against gravity. From the beginning, he only lifted light weights. When that became difficult, he lifted his arms over his head without weights and stretched to the ceiling as many times as he could. Persons, dealing with a neurological disease, should strive more for stamina than lifting for power. When my son worked as a trainer at a fitness center, he taught power lifting by lifting maximum weight 10 times. That may be a dangerous strategy when the muscles are no longer recuperating normally. Lifting to increase stamina entails working with a small amount of weight more than 10 repetitions. I do not recommend lifting so strenuously that muscles are sore the next day.

Repetition Helps Develop Coordination.

Dean would practice doing fine motor activities. He would wring out a wet dish cloth standing at the sink, throw and catch soft balls (sitting activity), bat balloons back and forth to me (sitting down), and open and close empty jars.

Practicing with his trumpet turned out to be one of the very best exercise activities that he did. Holding up his trumpet and working the fingers helped the stamina in his arms while building his breath control. His voice projection was actually normal during the year and half that he practiced on the trumpet.

Practice, Practice, Practice.

He picked up pennies with his fingertips and put them into a container. He colored pictures with markers or crayons, wrote notes in longhand, and wrote the grocery list. None of these tasks was easy, but Dean felt he needed to persevere.

A fun activity that we did together, worked on his arm function and his eye tracking abilities. I would sit in a chair about 10 feet away from him. We would each hold a big soft ball. Initially we threw one ball back and forth. On our adventurous days, Dean and I would toss our balls at the same time to the other person. Sometimes the balls would crash together and fly all over the room, but with practice we got fairly good at keeping the tosses going. He became so talented at our throwing game that we were able to toss two tennis balls back and forth. More often than not, we ended the session with some good laughing as I went around the room retrieving stray balls.

Implementing Adaptations For Daily Care Improves Independence.

Simple little adjustments can make a huge difference in the amount of help your loved one will need.

Dressing Oneself

We found that it was worth making the modifications that allowed Dean to continue to do as much for himself as possible. He was able to dress himself without a great deal of effort and frustration until the middle stage of the disease when he had trouble problem solving. Then it was easier for me to pick out clothes and help him dress. When zippers and buttons became too difficult, I ordered many pairs of khaki pants with elastic waists from an online company. They were about $10-12 and looked nice with an over hanging shirt. This allowed him to enter a men's restroom at church and be independent for several more months. When he began to use a cane for outings, the elastic waist bands were easier to manage and still maintain his balance. Naturally every person will have his own clothes preferences. For some, giving up the tailored look would be too much to ask.

For my husband, comfort was the first priority. Being less mobile, yet susceptible to temperature changes, Dean would need more warmth in the winter and less layers in the summer. I purchased several pairs of flannel pants and fleece shirts at a discount department store for winter wear. The elastic waist bands made them easy to get on and off. Shorts with elastic waist bands and big T-shirts made dressing especially easy in the summer. More roominess is necessary to get arms in sleeves when shoulders are painful or less mobile.

These are the clothing adjustments that worked for us:

Hats: After LBD, sunlight hurt Dean's eyes. We purchased a wide-brimmed cowboy hat on one of our vacations that went with us wherever we went. Suntan lotion was also very important for skin protection.

Shoes: I was very careful with the shoes that Dean wore. Sloppy slippers and floppy sandals can catch and trip a person. Dean had occasional swelling in his ankles and his feet were too sensitive to go barefooted. We had a variety of easy to don shoes depending on comfort, distance to walk, and fashion requirements. Around the house he wore soft, calf-leather moccasins that seemed to give him the best feel for the floor surface. When he wore dress pants, he wore a light-weight, soft leather black loafer with a sure-grip rubber sole. For longer distances or rough ground, he wore leather sneakers. Only the sneakers needed to be tied. Using a small shoe horn to ease his foot into any of the shoes helped. Shoe horns come in different sizes and lengths.

Socks: We used a variety of socks. The sensitivity in Dean's feet determined whether he wanted very thin or very thick socks. In the winter, he wore 100 percent wool socks that were soft, warm and very tolerable. We had three pairs that I rotated and hand washed. During days when he had swelling, I put support stockings on his feet. There is a slippery, silky socket device that is new since I struggled with putting the elastic hose on my husband's feet. It fits over the toes and along the bottom surface of the foot to the heel. The elastic stocking slips easily over the socket. Once in place, the socket can be pulled out and stored to be used the next time. If I could have videotaped the first time that I put support stockings on Dean's feet, I could have sold it to America's Funniest Home Videos for big money.

Shirts and Coats: Dean could best get into big loose coats that were roomy in the shoulders. Depending on shoulder flexibility, I might need to reach through the sleeve from the outside bottom of the sleeve toward the shoulder to grab his hand and pull the hand out the bottom. Bigger shirts or stretchy materials were easier to maneuver than smaller, tighter shirts. When one shoulder had less dexterity than the other, I started that arm through the sleeve first. I learned to give Dean a double check before we went out into public. Because of his vision and dexterity problems, he might not have the buttons lined up right. Occasionally his shorts or shirts would be inside out.

Underwear and pants: We had to break my husband's habit of taking his pants off while standing, which had become risky. We applied shorts either lying in bed or sitting on the edge of the bed. He pulled up the front, I did the back adjustment when necessary. To get his shorts to his waist when lying down, he needed to bend his knees, place feet flat on the bed, and lift his buttocks off the surface of the bed. When starting in sitting, I would monitor his balance as he stood and pulled the pants up to his waist. On particularly bad days, I would roll him side to side in the bed. We donned the pants in the same way. I needed to hem several pairs of his pants. With his stooped posture, his trouser legs would drag on the floor. I was afraid he would trip on the pants if I didn't hem them.

Buttons: Dean had difficulty lining up the buttons, both where to start and where to push the button through the hole. It was easier to pick clothes without buttons to wear. If a caregiver is handy with a sewing machine, Velcro strips work well on each side of the shirt opening. Sew the buttons onto the outside of the button hole and the shirt will look like it is buttoned.

Zippers: Most people with neurological diseases, motor weakness, and problems with finger dexterity will eventually have great difficulty manipulating zippers and belts. These tasks require coordination of both hands working on the zipper together. It is more challenging if the sensation in the fingers declines. Some men find that suspenders are a great alternative to belts.

Eating

Adjustments are a must! We improvised and modified everything to keep Dean feeding himself. Eating skills varied greatly throughout the course of Dean's disease. With the fluctuation in skills symptomatic of LBD, he could be independent one day and fully dependent the next. In fact, his eating skills in the later stages of the disease could vary widely from morning to night. Meals were more enjoyable and less demanding if I stayed prepared and flexible.

Spills Happen

In the middle phase of the disease, Dean began to have problems with spilling. He could initiate reaching for a cup or glass, get the container halfway to his mouth; and his hand would fall to his lap, spilling the fluid all over his front. This was, obviously, a messy problem but, more so, a demoralizing safety issue. Hot coffee fell in his lap causing a fairly large burn on one occasion. Anything in the hand obviously went flying when he lost control. Clean ups were easier when visiting at our son's house. He had three dogs that waited patiently by Grampa's chair at every meal. Following are several modifications that worked for us.

We covered the kitchen table with a plastic table cloth and plastic place mats. Either one was extended to protect his lap.

We put an area rug under the chair that could be flipped outside or washed in the washing machine.

I used the plastic joke bib at home that Dean got at his 70th birthday party. It kept his shirt clean. In a restaurant, we asked for more napkins to cover his lap.

Cups with lids prevented spills that could burn. Toddler cups worked for cold drinks and water.

He chose food entrees that he could eat more quickly and required less cutting. Pancakes were an anytime favorite. At home, I generally cut up all food into small bite-sized pieces. Slowness affected his eating in a restaurant.

I carried both plates to the table when we attended pot-luck suppers.

Choking

In the advanced stages of the disease, the throat muscles will begin to work much more slowly. Choking can become a serious problem. Certainly, food can get caught and block breathing. Inhaling small pieces of food or liquids into the windpipe and eventually into the lungs can be less obvious but just as serious. Food or liquids into the lungs is called aspiration and often leads to pneumonia and possibly death. If a person begins to choke regularly on sips of liquids or any food at meals, a swallowing test by a speech and language pathologist should be done. Your doctor would need to order the test. Should it be determined that aspiration is happening, the speech therapist or an occupational therapist can teach the caregiver feeding tips to avoid the choking. There are products that can be added to the liquids, even coffee, to thicken the liquids for safer swallowing. Meats can be ground to a paste form that is easier to maneuver in the mouth. Soft vegetables and fruits are preferable at this stage. Skins on apples, potatoes, and chicken should be removed before serving. Ice cream and puddings work well. And smaller bites will cause less choking.

Modifying Bathing Techniques Is a Critical Area of Concern.

Bathing

Bathing can be pleasurable or intolerable. It ranks high on the list of things to do to maintain good health and social acceptability; but, is equally high on the dangerous-activities list. Making the bathroom area free of clutter improves efficiency and safety.

Showers

In the early stage of the disease, I found that removing the shower doors and installing a rod and shower curtain gave much better access into and out of our walk-in shower. Adding a shower seat inside the shower and a hand-held shower nozzle was a bonus. When I needed to shampoo my husband's hair or help him wash, the hand held nozzle allowed me to direct the spray onto his hair and back while he was sitting. He was safe and comfortable. I stayed dry.

Falling is a real danger. Stability can be increased with strategically placed grab bars around the shower. There are several types available in hardware stores. We also used a good gripping mat inside all showers. I learned to take a rolled up mat with us on trips. Most shower stalls in hotels were too slippery.

Handing Dean a soapy wash cloth eliminated the danger he posed when he tried to bend over to pick up dropped soap. Caregivers need to be ever vigilant to avoid the risk of falls.

Burns in the shower are another concern. The short term memory issues prevented Dean from remembering which direction was hot and which cold. When I painted the shower wall with a BIG H and C, Dean was able to adjust water temperature without wearing his glasses. To be certain that he didn't inadvertently scald himself, I set the maximum water heater temperature at 140 degrees.

Getting safely out of the shower takes preparation as well. He was much easier to hold on to when he was dry. On days when he was fairly unstable, he sat on the shower chair and dried off. We always made sure that he did not step out of the shower with wet feet onto a wet slippery floor. That would have been as slippery as stepping on ice.

Bath Tub Bathing

If the home does not have a shower, preparations are needed early in the disease. It is easy to get into the tub. One day it may take the Emergency Medical Technician's to get a person out of the tub.

Most homes will accommodate a small tub bench that can fit over the side of the tub and extend into the tub. As long as a person can walk a few steps to sit onto the bench, tub baths are a feasible way to bathe. Medical supply stores have many varieties of tub benches. A physical therapist or occupational therapist will be able to give expert suggestions for accommodating all the equipment for the bathroom. The hand-held shower nozzle and grab bars are also helpful for tub bathing.

Bed Baths or Sponge Baths

When balance is too precarious to get safely into a shower or tub, a person will need to wash or be washed via a basin and cloth. On days when it is too much to get out of bed, bathing is still important. Supplies prearranged will help to expedite the bathing process. More information about organization will be presented in the next chapter.

Modifications Will Be Needed for All Self Care and Hygiene

Shaving and Hair Cuts

If a man is comfortable with an electric razor, he may be independent for a longer time than if he prefers a straight razor. He does not need as much dexterity in the wrists to use an electric razor. Dean liked a straight-razor cut. When he lost too much hand dexterity to cut around corners, it was easier and safer to grow a beard. The few times that I tried to shave him, he looked like he had tried to walk through a briar bush.

He also had his hair buzzed. Both helped to speed up hygiene in the mornings. I could clip his hair and beard easily once a week. Our Council on Aging agency would have sent out an aide to help Dean's shaving and showers during the week, but he felt he was managing fine with my help.

Tooth brushing

The emesis basin that is given to all persons in the hospital can also be very helpful at home. Sometimes Dean needed to sit on the bed and brush his teeth. He would be too tired and shaky to stand at the sink and brush. When dexterity in his arms and wrists decreased, we used an electric toothbrush. The tool did the work and got to all places in his mouth. After we started with the electric brush, his dentist noticed that Dean's gums were healthier.

Grooming toes and nails

Seeing a specialist for toenail care may be the best suggestion, especially if someone has a circulation problem. It only takes a tiny nip to start an infection in the foot that can be very difficult to heal.

Treating Dean to a pedicure was really a treat for both of us. We did afternoon pedicures followed by ice cream for several years.

When I did home grooming, I mimicked the salon techniques and started by soaking each foot in an astringent solution. We used inexpensive mouth wash or Epsom salts before I began the clipping. If home grooming is preferred, the caregiver should be diligent about soaking the utensils in alcohol or mouth wash after each use. Foot fungus spreads easily.

Summary

Changes in coordination will definitely affect how a spouse manages daily care tasks. I certainly encouraged Dean to do as much as he could for himself for as long as he possibly could, because I knew it helped stimulate his thinking and problem solving skills. His independent efforts, however, were not always easier on me.

One morning, he was happily showering by himself as I stood at the sink fully dressed, brushing my teeth. It was indeed a shock to be deluged with a steady flow of water, over the top of the shower curtain from the hand held nozzle. As I yelped and turned to see what he was doing, he proceeded to drench the pictures and mirror by the sink in his effort to get the nozzle head shut off.

He thought my soaking was hilariously funny.

Chapter 8

A Place for Everything and Everything in Its Place

A right time to plant and another to reap,
—Ecclesiastes 3:2 The Message

This chapter will address many tips for proactively organizing the house and car. In the early phase of the disease, simple tricks can allow the spouse to stay independent without safety concerns. In the middle and later stages, when more help is needed, the care can be more efficient and less laborious for the caregiver if all supplies are arranged in easy-to-reach containers. This was a huge piece of the success story for us. It may take cleaning out clutter and rearranging furniture, but the results are worth the effort.

During the years that I did home health as a PT, I saw horrendous living arrangements with extensive clutter, minimal space to walk, and piles of junk stashed in corners. Fortunately, I also saw the positive set ups where the family and caregivers had made the effort to plan, organize, and structure the environment to accommodate for the caregiving needs. Care was so much easier for everyone in the organized homes.

For the first two years after Dean retired, I worked several days of the week, and he took care of the house. When he couldn't remember which buttons to push on the appliances, I marked stove, washer, dryer, and dishwasher with arrows to jog his memory. I wrote out instructions for the DVD and marked the remote control with a rubber band so Dean's buddies could play a DVD when I was not home. These minor adjustments kept Dean and our home operating smoothly.

All that I did in our home may not be feasible in someone else's home. The importance of this chapter is encouraging caregivers to plan ahead to be ready for any care need BEFORE the need becomes an emergency.

Bathroom

"Containerize" Supplies

It isn't always possible, but if a dedicated bathroom is available with all materials at fingertip reach, it would assist the caregiver. Just as mothers set up the changing area for an infant, caregivers need to have supplies available and within quick reach to care for a person with limited balance.

I put a shelf box on the wall over the commode to keep many supplies handy. It wasn't pretty, but it held rubber/latex gloves, q-tips, emesis basis for teeth brushing, shampoos, extra bars of soap and wet wipes.

In a small plastic box on the sink, I kept a straw, comb, water cup, and razor. The items on the sink were duplicated in his tote bag for overnight outings.

The wash basin we brought home from the hospital fit nicely under the sink, readily available for bed-bath-days.

A basket on the top of the commode held a stack of small old towels that I used for easy clean ups. In another basket, I kept old washcloths.

Cleaning supplies needed their own designated corner and bucket.

Bathroom Equipment

An elevated commode seat is tremendously valuable when strength in the legs decreases, making it much easier to stand up and sit down. There are many types available in medical supply stores that are easy to install. I purchased one with four legs that fit over the commode. It had arms for security. This one had a bucket attachment and could be used as a bedside commode. Unfortunately, the armrests provided a false sense of safety. To help prevent tipping, I placed weights on the legs to increase stability.

Grab bars would increase safety around the commode. Some therapists recommend installing a medical Super Pole from floor to ceiling instead of grab bars. When installed properly, the pole is very sturdy, and is safer to pull on when attempting to stand up.

Caregivers should consider that at some point in the progression of the disease, physical assisting will be needed to help the person get on and off the commode, in and out of the bath area. With that in mind, space around the commode and shower/tub should be sufficiently cluttered free to allow two people in that area together.

Bedroom

Clear Out and Organize

Convenience and hygiene are considerations for the ease of the caregiver. Comfort, rest, and safety are important considerations for the loved one. Taking the time to set up the bedroom will be a tremendous help and make things easy to manage throughout all stages of the disease.

Clear out clutter to provide as much open floor space as possible. Twice the amount of floor space is needed in a handicap bedroom to store walker, wheelchair, and any other equipment. The walking path from hallway to bathroom to bed needs to be wide enough for two people to walk side by side. Falls can happen when the caregiver does not have sufficient room to provide walking assistance. Falls can cause serious injuries if someone hits a table or other furniture edge on the way to the floor.

A place for everything and everything in its place! This type of organization will help immensely if the caregiver has to come in for a 4:00 AM emergency clean up. I cleared out a corner of our clothes closet, and put the cedar chest into the closet to increase bedroom floor space. Then, I put all the paper products for incontinence on the chest. This arrangement helped me keep track of our supply inventory. I knew immediately when I was nearly out of the padded night-time briefs.

Clean sheets, pillow cases, and protector pads for Dean's bed were stored above the paper products. This also helped keep track of the clean supply. When the number of protector pads was low, I knew I needed to wash clothes.

"I Can't Lose This!" items: Dean became very anxious if he couldn't find his glasses, keys, or wallet with insurance cards. Eventually, all these items went into a fanny pack and were kept by the front door. In the early phase, we needed a dedicated basket or drawer.

The "See it and use it" wall hooks: Dean was able to pick out his own clothes easily if he could see them. I screwed a set of hooks by the closet door for all his favorite clothes. I would hang his shorts and shirts in plain sight.

Night stand items that were used every night were in a basket by the bed. All of these items were duplicated in the tote bag packed for vacations.

Soiled clothing had its own basket in the corner, very obvious to Dean. If he could see the basket for dirty clothes, he would place items in the receptacle. Opening the closet door to find the basket didn't work with the LBD.

Waste paper items went into a separate large vinyl waste container with a plastic garbage bag liner in another corner.

Bed Set up

Sleeping disorders are common for persons with LBD. Adequate sleep for both the caregiver and the patient is vital. If the person sleeps well throughout the night, the caregiver may also be able to get good uninterrupted sleep. We sought solutions to keep Dean in his bed all night and more importantly, asleep all night.

A clock with lighted digital numbers was placed on a table easily visible during the night. At night, Dean could see the clock, realize it was still night, and go back to sleep.

Rails fitted to the bed provided a support to help him transfer from lying down to sitting up and greatly helped protect his shoulders. More importantly, they provided some protection to keep him safely in bed at night.

Blankets need to provide adequate warmth. During the late stage of the disease, Dean was not able to pull covers over his body and could not regulate his body temperature well. I used a layering system of light to heavy and added more as the temperature outside warranted. On very cold nights during the winter, I used flannel sheets that immediately gave him a sense of warmth when he got into bed. If he was cold, he might or might not call me, but he would definitely be restless and yell out all night. We both slept better if I could anticipate the type of blanket mix that he needed.

Protective coverings are vinyl mattress covers, washable rubber sheet protectors, and paper liners that keep sheets dry if someone is incontinent during the night. I used all three because I didn't want to get up in the middle of the night and change wet sheets. I used extra absorbent pads inside the large disposable diapers. I kept trying different brands and different combinations until I found the products and the combination that kept everything inside the pads all night long. Many pharmacists will work with the caregiver to stock any night time supplies. Just ask if a particular product can be ordered on a regular basis.

A video baby monitor worked well during the advanced stage of the disease. Dean didn't always call me when he needed help or was attempting to get out of bed by himself. The screen would alert me to his safety needs. Our brand had a screen that could go from room to room with me.

Alternative Bed Arrangements

Some families may choose to use the chair recliner for night time sleeping. This has benefits and disadvantages. It is certainly easier to transfer someone into and out of the lift chair rather than the bed. One negative involves the position of the hips and knees in the chair. Most chairs do not fully recline. While in the chair the hips and knees are always slightly flexed. Over time, the last few degrees of extension will become restricted. This will cause the person to stand and walk with a bend in the hips and knees similar to the bend maintained while sleeping in the chair. If chair sleeping is the choice, caregivers might discuss ways that the person can exercise the hips and knees during the day to maintain full range of motion in the hips and knees.

A second negative involves hygiene. If a person becomes incontinent, the chair will become soiled during the night and develop an odor. I would recommend reading the section on bed set up to gain tips on protecting the surface of the chair with protective pads.

Many families will need a hospital bed in their home at some point. Advantages are many. The mattress is moisture proof. The entire bed can be raised or lowered to make transferring easier. Bed care at the proper height for the caregiver protects her back. Some restraint is built in with rails the length of the bed. Also, hospital beds can be equipped with other equipment to accommodate more medical needs.

Leisure Area

The main seating area to watch TV should be set up for easy access to supplies. Seating should be comfortable and protected with rubber pads. Dean used a lift chair for two years as his primary place to sit. The lift chair is a stuffed leisure chair that has a hydraulic mechanism to recline the back or lift the seat into the air as a help when a person is trying to stand up out of the chair. It was meant for independent transfers in and out of the chair, but didn't work quite that way for Dean. He could only work the buttons correctly 50 percent of the time. It served as a help for me to get him out of the chair; I pushed his buttons for him.

Before we purchased the lift chair, I put a second foam cushion in a padded chair to elevate the seat. It was much easier for my tall husband to push up out of the higher seat.

Since the loved one will be spending a significant amount of time sitting in a lounge chair, supplies should be containerized around the chair as recommended for the bedroom and bathroom. We put a basket and table next to Dean's chair that held his magazines, tissues, water bottle, plastic trash bag, and any other items he might need regularly. Our TV remote was always hiding somewhere in our family room. It became much easier to find when I put a strip of shocking red duct tape on one side of it.

Simple Modifications When Away from the House

Ramps are necessary if there are steps to get into the home. There are handicap codes established for safety that should be followed if the family builds their own ramp. The incline should measure at least one foot in length for every 1 inch in elevation. Some city codes may be different. Portable ramps made of light weight aluminum can be very helpful for one or two steps into a house. They can be folded up, carried easily, and transported in a large car or van.

Car and Community Adaptations

Some suggestions are listed under Traveling by Car in Chapter 4.

A handicap sticker served us very well. It is easy to obtain in our state. We took a medical statement signed by the doctor to the bureau of motor vehicle office and paid a small fee.

Limitations on driving will be crucially important at some point. There will come a time when driving a car is no longer an option for someone with the mental and physical limitations of LBD. The family must assess carefully, and keys must be taken. No one wants to be told they are unfit to drive, and certainly no loving family member wants to enter into that discussion with a spouse or an ailing parent. It will require big changes in daily care if the ailing person relies on the car for grocery shopping or medical appointments. Options must be found. In all of the neuromotor diseases, coordination is compromised. Reactions become slower. Vision may not be accurate for either acuity or normal field of vision. And lastly, mental judgment and processing may be impaired.

A family member does not have to be medically trained to be able to determine when to pull the keys. Watch for the lack of neck flexibility needed to see traffic in the other lane. Note hand strength and the ability to turn the wheel quickly or fully. It can be easier on the caregiver if they enlist the help of the medical doctor or the adult children. They can tell the loved one that driving is no longer an option because of the disease, with an authority that is difficult to challenge. Keys may still need to be hidden. Driving abilities may be more difficult to assess with LBD than with some other diseases because of the waxing and waning aspect. Being proactive is safest. Dean was losing his bearings in the grocery store; he would eventually be lost on familiar streets. I realized he was not seeing accurately in the middle stage of the disease when I followed him home from tennis one night. He continuously rode the yellow line on an unlighted highway and did not move right when cars approached from the other direction.

As a positive, insurance rates should go down with only one driver. It was worth asking for us.

Car Maintenance

When the man of the house develops a long- term illness, car maintenance problems are yet another issue for his wife to handle. Traveling with a person with medical challenges is stressful enough, without dealing with a breakdown on the highway.

My motto has always been to prevent a problem whenever possible, before a problem needed to be fixed. After one breakdown on the highway, I traded in both of our older cars that did not have warranties, and bought a new car that had a 100,000 mile warranty. With the deal, I also got roadside service benefits and valet service for regular maintenance check-ups. The dealership would come to my home, leave me a loaner car, drive back to the service center, and return my car later in the day. This would not have been part of the package if I had not negotiated the benefit and received a signed letter of that service. I needed the availability of transportation which a loaner car provided. With the purchase, I also acquired a team of service people that we trusted. Car maintenance became a matter of watching for the expiration date on the windshield.

Summary

This is certainly not an exclusive list. The idea I want to convey is that problems can often be solved with some keen thinking, good suggestions, and inexpensive supplies. At times a modification can restore full independence for a longer time. Learning to watch how the subtle changes are evolving will also allow the caregiver to be proactive for safety in the home. I had to curtail use of the stove when Dean would forget to turn the burners off, or would turn on the wrong burner. He stopped carrying a credit card when he misplaced the card on an outing with our daughter, and the card had to be cancelled. Instead I gave him a $20 bill to buy lunch or ice cream for the grandchildren. He still carried a key to the house on a chain, but all identifying information was removed from the chain. If he lost the key, it was just a key.

He stopped answering the phone when he was unable to write down the messages. He should have stopped answering the door before he ordered several magazines that we didn't read!

Living with someone with declining functional skills is like learning to dance. Sometimes you lead and sometimes you follow. Sometimes you get your toes stepped on. Eventually you and your partner master the basics of moving together; you get into the flow. Garth Brooks sang in *The Dance* that if he had known ahead that he would get his heart broken after the Big Dance, he could have avoided the pain by not attending. But, he also would have missed the elation he felt while dancing with a special person.[24]

Chapter 9

All Senses Can be Affected

and a time to dance;
—Ecclesiastes 3:4 RSV

What does "sensory" mean? The sensory system of the body gathers information about the outside world and sends that information to our brains. The brain makes sense of the sensory signals and determines whether to ignore them or do something with the information. Most people will be able to tolerate wearing jewelry. Our brains know we are wearing rings, but say, "No big deal". For some people, when their hair begins to touch the collar; it signals time to get a hair cut.

Our sensory system is of great value. It is often our protector. When a child learns that too much heat can cause pain, he shies away from an oven. When he learns that gravity causes things to fall downward, he will be more careful on stairs. We need our senses.

Unfortunately in LBD, the sensory messages that the body sends to the sensory area of the brain are often not interpreted accurately. The eyes may see that a step is seven inches high. If the brain doesn't register the height of seven inches, it may direct the foot to only step up a height of four inches. Obviously, Mr. Foot will bump into the stair step rather than clearing it. The person attached to the foot will probably fall forward with a confused look upon his face. Conversely, if the flower pattern in the carpet is perceived as 3- dimensional, a person will lift the foot very high to step over imagined flowers. The senses that most people recognize are hearing, sight, taste, and smell. More important to overall function are the senses of touch, movement, and awareness of the body in space (proprioception). The senses of sight and smell tell us that a cup of coffee in is front of us. The senses of touch and proprioception tell us to be very careful when picking up and drinking a hot cup of coffee.

For many years of my working career, I was a school physical therapist and worked with children who had learning problems. My job was to help them better use all their senses and even quiet some of the senses that were hyper. When I could accomplish this for each child, he or she would be able to concentrate, focus and actually learn better in school. In many ways, my husband resembled the children I had worked with in the school systems.

When I began looking for information about LBD on the internet, sensory dysfunction was listed as a symptom. But the website did not elaborate on how the senses might become dysfunctional or what techniques might be available to work with any sensory malfunctions. Unfortunately, all Dean's senses malfunctioned at one time or another. We worked hard to support what was working to give him a better sense of his surroundings.

Touch: Normal and Abnormal

Some people are hypersensitive and some are hyposensitive. Most people do not feel the clothes on their skin. But there are some people who can't wear wool next to their skin because it feels itchy or prickly. People who are hyposensitive may say they have a high threshold for pain. All of these reactions are within normal limits

The touch part of the brain can play tricks. Some people who have had a foot or leg removed, still "feel" the foot itch or hurt. Amputees call this phantom pain. For other people, the nerves to a body part stop delivering effective touch sensations to the brain. Doctors call this neuropathy. Healthy people experience this when a foot "falls asleep". A foot or hand can become numb if the circulation somehow becomes impeded. The feeling of prickly pain that the person experiences when the circulation returns to the foot or hand, is typical of what someone with a neuropathy might feel. This was the case for my husband. His feet always felt prickly. He could not walk on some of our carpet barefooted because the sensation from the carpet fibers felt like needles. This uncomfortable sensation only lasts a few minutes when touch is normal. It was a constant problem for Dean.

Although neuropathy is not listed as a typical symptom of LBD in the medical literature, it was a concurrent diagnosis for Dean and very annoying. I needed to be very gentle when handling his feet.

Dean experienced a strange form of sensation in his hands as well. He described it as feeling weird "gunk" on his hands and between his fingers. Sometimes he described it as grit on the fingers, sometimes strings that he could also "see" stretched out from his fingers. Nothing I could say would convince him that he did not have something in his hands. I would periodically reach out and let him place his gunk in my hand. He would then use his whole hand for awhile.

Some sensory techniques that I used with my students worked for Dean for short periods of time, but since the nerves/brain connection in his hands and feet was faulty, any long term effort was futile.

Deep pressure through the hands turned off the gunky feel. I would have him place his hands on the table and lean into the palms, then rock back in forth over his hands. When he was not steady enough to stand on his feet, I would push my palm into the palm of his hand while he was sitting. This was a good activity when we were spending time together in front of the TV.

I used warm wash cloths to wash the fingers and hands frequently, knowing that normally dirty hands would feel excessively dirty. When I dried them with a fluffy towel, I would rub them a little bit roughly to get the circulation moving into his hands. I also let him wear gloves if that helped on a particular day.

Exercise with his arms (raising his hands over his head, and lifting small weights) all helped. I moved his fingers around in gentle range of motion movements. Initially, the exercise with his fingers might have felt a bit uncomfortable, but his hands felt somewhat normal after we were done. None of these activities should cause pain.

I did not work on his feet as much as his hands because touch was more painful. I did move his toes up and down to be sure that he had the proper range of motion to be able to walk safely.

Hearing: Normal and Abnormal

Normally, the sensors in the ear pick up sound vibrations and change those vibrations into electrical signals that trigger the hearing center of the brain. When the brain receives each electrical signal it has the ability to recognize what object created that sound vibration. We hear a tinkling and recognize the sound came from a bell. Problems can arise in many older people because the ear mechanics breakdown. Hearing aids may be of help if the problem is in the ear. If the breakdown is in the brain area that interprets the sound waves coming in, it may appear as if someone is hard of hearing. In this instance; however, hearing aids generally do not help.

Background noise became a problem that bothered both of us. Crying children in a restaurant, loud commercials on TV, or many people talking in a crowded room would shut Dean down. He couldn't talk because he couldn't think past the room noise. On some nights, when we were watching a program on TV, he would forget what we were watching if we sat through all the commercials. I learned to mute all the commercials, so we could talk about the show we were watching. It worked even better to tape our favorite shows and skim through the commercials very fast.

Taste and Smell: Normal and Abnormal

When Dean's taste buds stopped working normally, he continued to enjoy eating but couldn't taste the food well. This may or may not have been an early symptom of the disease. Nothing in any of the treatment medications helped his taste return. I suspected that if Dean had lost his ability to taste, spicy foods might be better. Not so. He seemed to enjoy salt and pepper, but not other spices.

Changes in Dean's ability to smell things were interesting. During the middle stages of the disease, Dean's sense of smell increased dramatically. When we attended a new church, he became nauseated both of the first weeks we attended. We had to leave in the middle of the sermon both weeks to get him away from the sanctuary. The third week we sat on the far side of the church, in the last row. Amazingly, he was fine. I hadn't detected any odors on either side of the church.

That particular summer, he was very sensitive to warm air and outdoor smells as well. He could get nauseated just walking past an open door of a restaurant, for example. If I wore perfume, he might gag.

As hypersensitive to smells as he became in the middle phase of his disease, he was radically hyposensitive to smells latter. At one time, he couldn't smell his own body odors and didn't seem to care if he needed to bathe. This was a radical change for him. He had always been a clean freak.

Some of my home health patients became averse to bathing. Families might need to cajole to get them to bathe. I didn't have to go that far with Dean. He was willing to bathe if I scheduled it into his day. He just didn't recognize the need.

Sight: Normal and Abnormal

The ability to see accurately is extremely important. It affects all movements with the hands; all balance reactions when walking, and all feeling of normalcy in the environment. When a person becomes car sick to the point of nausea, it helps to sit in the front seat where the eyes can see the road. Vision works like hearing. If the eyes have a mechanical problem, glasses might help. If the vision center of the brain is dysfunctional, no treatment is available to fix the brain. Normally the brain interprets the information so that the muscles can act on that information. "Where are my keys? Oh, there are my keys."

The best word to describe Dean's vision on some days was quizzical. How he saw things was a mystery to me. For one span of time, if I did not constantly move him closer to the table, he would drop food into his lap. After a few bites, he would push back from the table and continue to reach across a gulley to spear his food. Naturally, he would drop pieces and, if I didn't stop him, he would lean out of his chair to retrieve the dropped pieces. It was as if he could see better from a distance than up close. He certainly could spot the droppings on the floor easily. Any dog would have thought he had landed in Heaven if he lived at our house during that time.

We began to notice visual disturbances in the middle stages of the disease. Dean complained of difficulty with depth perception on the tennis court. His eyes worked slower to track objects coming at him, such as moving tennis balls. It didn't help that his reflexes were also slowing down. I realized it was vision when he also had trouble determining how far away other cars were on the road. I had to take away his driving privileges when he pulled in front on oncoming cars twice in a one mile trip. Luckily, in both situations, the cars had a free lane to pull around him. I was afraid the next time might be disastrous.

He had ups and downs with his ability to read. He complained that his eyes might jerk when he was reading. It made it difficult for him to follow a line of print. He probably had jerking with his eyes the way he had jerking with his hands when trying to hold the paper still. We stopped our subscriptions to magazines because he felt the pictures were too busy. New glasses didn't help his acuity problems. That was evidenced around the house and out in the community as well. Fortunately, when I would explain what he was really looking at, he could refocus and make out the true pattern. He could actually tell me on some days that his vision was fuzzy.

One summer he was seeing double much of the time. We noticed this as he was watching a tennis match on television. He wondered why they were playing with three balls on the court. His startled remark was, "Is that legal?"

The technicians in the optometrist' office would adjust the fit of Dean's glasses for free. This was a wonderful service in the later stages as Dean would lie down on his glasses, remove them with a one hand pull, or leave them in unsafe places. Even if his eyes had worked well, he couldn't have seen clearly with the bent frames.

Strategies to Help with Vision Changes

As with the hallucinations, discussed in Chapter 2, all I could do was explain as gently as possible that what his eyes were telling him was not real. My husband had a placid personality and accepted the limitations without a great deal of anger. For many people, vision problems can be extremely frustrating and unnerving. It can be easier to just sit in one spot and not have to deal with depth perception needed for walking either in the home or in more taxing situations outside of the home.

I gave Dean the opportunity to continue reading but didn't expect him to remember what he read. When we were trying to enjoy a book, I read to him. If we played a game, I kept his score as well as mine.

It took courage, but I took away the keys to the car when I realized his impaired vision made driving unsafe.

As needed, I used direct hands-on support when he was on his feet. I needed to hang on tight when he walked up a step because he no longer judged true depth.

The Sense of Movement is also Called the Vestibular System.

Normally, the part of the ear called the semi-circular canals gathers information about the position of the head. As the brain monitors the head position, it can determine where the body is in space and how fast it is moving. Picture the fluid bubble inside of a level tool that indicates when the level is straight and not tipped more in one direction than another. The fluid inside the ear labyrinth does the same thing. If the head is tipped too far in one direction, the brain alarms go off and the body adjusts to prevent a fall. The movement centers are extremely important for all balance reactions and body awareness. Balance is the simplest function of the vestibular system.

The most complicated function is monitoring all the other senses mentioned above. It is like the traffic cop directing traffic on a busy corner. It somehow senses all the information coming into the brain from all sensory channels, determines what is important and what is not. It is the vestibular system that helps us make the decisions about all the motor movements in our every-day life. "OK, I know you are hungry, cold, have to go to the bathroom, and you are late for work. Go to the bathroom first, then….."

What we school therapists found as we treated school-aged children with vestibular problems was that all the senses were linked to the balance and movement centers of the vestibular system. If we could improve balance, the child's reading and memory improved. Their emotions normalized and their focus improved. Often the touch system would become more normal. Knowing that, Dean and I worked on balance every chance we could.

Strategies to Help Balance in the Early Stages:

Walking is not just getting from one place to another. Walking stimulates the vestibular system of the body and helps all of the senses work better. These are some of the activities Dean did in his physical therapy exercise program that require a trained therapist to implement.

Balancing on a big therapy ball helped him improve his equilibrium and balance reactions.

Balancing on his hands and knees activated the vestibular system in a horizontal position.

Rolling on a mat from the back, to side, to belly with help, as needed, improved everything. It was a wonderful exercise for Dean. It helped him continue to roll over by himself in bed.

He used equipment in the clinic called Pilates that helped maintain movement of his arms and legs.

When on vacations, he practiced floating on his back and on his belly in pools. This was extremely difficult to do in the later stages. If I did not hold him, he wouldn't have been able to correct himself in the water and could have drowned. Exercise in the water seemed to help his balance when he was out of the pool.

Strategies in the Later Stages:

We practiced movement awareness in our home in the following ways:

We continued walking using the walker. I put low weighted cuffs on his ankles to give him a better sense of where his feet were. I used gait belts for safety and continued to walk him around the house during the day.

We danced together in the family room, especially working on backward and sideways movements, and turning in space.

We continued to practice getting down to a floor mat and getting back up. This may not be feasible without a therapist present.

When sitting, I encouraged him to reach out, up, away from the body to stretch his back and arms and to open his chest and expand his lung volume. If he couldn't stretch his arms out fully, I helped him stretch as much as his arms would stretch.

I don't think insurance policies pay for the medical benefits of a cruise, but we noticed that while on each of the three cruises, his balance improved the longer he was on the ship. At the end of an eleven day cruise, he was actually able to play ping pong on the ship with good balance reactions and good hand movements. Maybe if we had lived on a ship for the next several years, he would have had less neurological degeneration. Just a thought…

Proprioception or Position of Body Parts in Space

Normal and Abnormal

When eyes are closed, healthy people can move an extended arm out from the side of the body to touch the tip of the nose. Sports analysts commend a basketball player for his ability to repeatedly shoot a three-point shot or to make consecutive free throws. These movements require a good sense of proprioception, knowing where our body parts are in space and being able to repeat specific movements.

A watch-repair specialist needs a different sense of proprioception than does the basketball player. Each needs to work extensively to train their bodies to work in precise movement patterns.

My husband lost any sense of where he was in space during one down phase of the disease. When he was standing, he could not turn, sit, or get into bed easily because he lost the awareness of the back of his body. If he could not see it, it did not exist. It was very difficult for him to take steps sideways or backward. He needed much physical prompting to walk even a few steps backward. He was as afraid of a step backward as he would have been of walking a tightrope high in the air.

He even lost the ability to recognize what vertical was. When he stood, he leaned backward rather than coming up and over his legs. Telling him to stand more upright didn't help. He thought he was standing upright. Even I had difficulty transferring him from one chair to another during those days.

Strategies to Help the Sense of Proprioception

There are many techniques to help proprioception problems. I used all of these strategies with the "clumsy" children who I treated in the schools. Initially, they would bump into other children when walking down the halls, trip on the stairs, and fall off the playground equipment. These little children also had very poor handwriting that was affecting school performance. Other associated problems were poor organization skills, poor memory retention, and limited focusing abilities.

This also described my husband's coordination. For the children, their brains had not fully developed the coordination skills: their "glass was half full". I helped them fill up their glasses with more coordination skills. The coordination loss for my husband was more like a hole in the bucket. His coordination reserves were draining away. I couldn't fix his problem, but I could help his brain remember how to do better what it used to do well.

Activities

When his balance was good, we continued to hit tennis balls. He also enjoyed miniature golf, shuffleboard, and playing billiards.

We played catch through all stages of the disease. When standing became unsafe, we did these activities sitting down. I batted balloons to him and he batted them back to me.

He marched around the house with high-stepping feet in all directions: forward, sideways, and backward. A safer way to do this is to march at the kitchen sink. If not at the sink, support with a gait belt is needed.

He stretched rubber bands apart with his fingers.

He stretched therapeutic bands in all directions with his hands and arms.

After doing some big-muscle exercise such as marching or throwing, we worked on coloring pictures inside the lines with crayons or colored pencils. He also practiced picking up pennies and putting them in the slot of a piggy bank. Making playdoh animals was fun with our grandchildren as well as therapeutic for Dean.

At home we worked on big muscles by dancing in the family room. He had to try to keep his feet moving to the beat of the music.

I encouraged him to do all of his own care activities that his level of ability allowed: zipping his coat, buttoning some of his buttons, turning the pages of the newspaper, washing his own body with a soapy cloth. Each of these tasks forced him to work the propriception areas of his brain. With each effort, he was exercising his brain. I didn't expect success with every activity.

Therapists always say, "If you don't use it, you lose it." Working with the sensory system and the balance reactions, we tried to preserve the thinking and motor parts of the brain. We did some variation of all the activities listed in this chapter through all phases of the disease. Some of these activities will require implementation by a therapist after an evaluation.

Chapter 10

All Systems of the Body Can be Affected by the Disease

a time to cast away stones, and a time to gather stones together;.
—Ecclesiastes 3:5 RSV

Lewy Body Dementia can create problems with many systems of the body, not just the nervous system. Although the damage sites are in the brain, effects can be seen in most other parts of the body. What we discuss in this chapter are some of the lesser mentioned problems that can be as difficult to live with as the dementia and the loss of balance. In fact, some can make life miserable until solutions are found to remedy the problems.

It is confusing to have so many problems that seem unrelated, yet originate from a strange disease process. If Dean did not have LBD, he wouldn't have had constipation and nausea problems. His cuts healed just fine before he was diagnosed with LBD. He had no unusual problems with his eyes. And certainly he had no problems with breathing or stamina. In fact, he could play two hours of tennis in hot sun before the LBD symptoms kicked-in.

There are typical age-related problems: the joints (arthritis), heart (blood pressure), and vision (glaucoma). This is not what this chapter discusses. All of these problems have diseased tissue or mechanical problems specifically in the organs. Any of these conditions will require medical attention not related to the LBD management. My husband had no other medical problems and took no other prescriptions before he was originally diagnosed with the PD and then the LBD.

Understanding the interweaving of LBD in all the systems of the body, should help caregivers be better prepared and proactive in management. Any problem or complication should be discussed with the doctors managing the ongoing LBD. A strange symptom may be part of the LBD picture in a round-a-bout way. It may be related to drugs that are prescribed. The importance is to understand that LBD can affect how everything in the body works.

Cardio Pulmonary/ Heart, Circulatory, and Lung Systems

Blood Pressure

Regulating Dean's blood pressure became one of his most debilitating issues. The doctors could not be sure if the fluctuating blood pressure was a side effect of medications that were treating the dementia; or if it was a symptom of the disease. Pressure could jump to 200/90 (which is dangerously high) or fall drastically to 90/60 and cause fainting and falls. Luckily, the lower pressures were the most common and could be treated with a drug that was supposed to stabilize the pressure. I didn't like to have Dean fainting whenever he stood, but at least the lower end would not likely cause a heart attack or a stroke.

We bought an electric blood pressure measuring device that was very easy to apply and read. Most drug stores will carry them. All I had to do was put the cuff on Dean's arm and push a button. We kept a notebook next to the device where I jotted down his pressures. The notebook went with us for Dean's doctor visits to help the doctors understand what his pressure was doing while he was at home.

As long as the blood pressure is unstable and your loved one is fainting when he stands; walking will need to be closely supervised or possibly discontinued. Orthostatic hypotension is the term used to describe the sudden fall in blood pressure when a person stands up. Fainting or becoming dizzy when standing is definitely a condition to share with the doctors. Pressure should be neither too high nor too low.

The first time we observed this in my husband, was when Dean rose out of a chair to say good-bye to our son-in-law. He walked to the foyer and began to fall over backward like a tree in the forest. Luckily, my son-in-law and I caught him and eased him to the floor. As soon as he was on the floor and horizontal; he looked at us, smiled, and asked what he was doing on the floor.

Dean learned to interpret how his body was reacting to the blood pressure fluctuations. He would get a twitch or a jerk and feel dizzy. Those twitches taught him to sit down immediately. This is a vitally important point for those with LBD. There may be signs, like Dean's twitching, that can warn you that something bad is about to happen. A caregiver needs to be ever watchful for strange reactions.

It seemed that Dean had more problems with blood pressure after a big meal. We learned to take the wheelchair into a restaurant in anticipation of an episode after he had eaten. He learned that a quick nap after a big meal worked best.

Once he started to take the medication to regulate the low blood pressure, he was much safer. During the weeks it took to regulate the appropriate dosage, Dean wore elastic support hose. I wish I could say the medication worked wonderfully, but it didn't. I never fully trusted his ability to wander in the house alone anymore. Medication and the support hose helped to stabilize the bouts of pressure dropping, but I was always suspicious that the pressure would drop when he stood; and he would fall and break a bone.

Fatigue

Stamina and fatigue problems are expected with LBD and PD. Dean had problems with both. Exercise seemed to fill his energy bucket. Naps helped a little, but never gave him a fully rested feeling. He could wake from a full night of sleep and still feel fatigued.

In the middle stage of the disease, his breathing tended to be shallow. This certainly contributed to his stamina issues. When we went for walks around the house, I had to remind him to take deep breaths. During the later phase, Dean tended to pant breathe all the time similar to the breathing that a women does during labor. After I reminded him to take deeper breaths, he would be okay for a short time, but then he would start to pant again. He needed to take purposeful deep breaths each time he attempted to stand and walk.

We practiced deep breathing. Dean would lie on the bed while I would coach him to breathe in through his nose and out through his mouth while he was doing the breathing exercise. A deep breath should raise the belly in an outward direction. The middle ribs should flair outward, and the upper chest should move in a lifting direction. We could notice better voice projection after the breathing exercises. He developed the ability to call for me anywhere in the house.

Again, I emphasize that any strange breathing pattern should be reported to the doctor.

Immune System

Sinus Infections

It was not uncommon to require two or three refills of an antibiotic to clear up his recurring sinus infections. A sinus infection for my husband wasn't just a runny nose. Any infection wiped him out until I could get him on an antibiotic. He would become mentally disoriented, extremely confused, and very weak physically. During those times, Dean needed to be on bed rest for two or three days.

His reaction to an infection was very bizarre. His severe mental confusion and disorientation might have looked to others as if the LBD had progressed to a new level of involvement. Amazingly, as soon as he would start the antibiotic, the mental clarity would return. Within another day, his physical abilities to transfer and walk would return. I witnessed this transformation so many times that I became a believer in what the antibiotic pills could do in my husband's situation.

Working in nursing homes has taught me that nurses are well trained to suspect an infection if an older person suddenly becomes confused and weakened. Caregivers, as well, might benefit from watching for any type of an infection in their loved one.

Healing Skin Abrasions

People with LBD may find that skin wounds do not heal quickly. Dean bumped his leg on a cement wall walking into our granddaughter's school one day. It was a very small scrape, but I was still treating that scrape four months later. At one point, it looked red and angry. That was an indication that it was becoming infected. Any open area needs to be shown to the doctor as soon as possible after you notice that the wound is not healing.

Small open areas should not be ignored. If an area becomes infected, it can lead to serious problems and spread throughout the body. It can become a life threatening situation. As you begin to treat a small scrape, it is a good idea to mark the outside of the open area with a pen so that you can see whether the injured area is shrinking.

All skin should be monitored regularly for abrasions. Sores can occur on arms, legs, or toes by bumping against furniture or hard surfaces. Skin abrasions should normally heal in two weeks. If healing is taking longer than that, it would be good to inform the doctor. Regular medical checks on open skin areas might be needed.

It is not uncommon for people with LBD to develop red crusty skin patches on the face above the eyes. Dean had other patches on the arms and legs and occasionally on his back. The rash on the face was listed on the LBD association website. These patchy areas could cause an itching problem, to the extent that he would scratch until he bled.

Any time that he opened the skin by scratching, I needed to cleanse it with an astringent. Your doctor may have a suggestion to heal the opened skin rashes and stop the itching.

The way a person sleeps can be important when preventing openings on the skin. If sleeping is always in the same position, the skin over boney areas can become sore. These areas need to be checked carefully: the tailbone, the heels, the ankle bones, and the elbows. If a person always sleeps on his side, the tailbone won't be a problem, but the hip and ankle will be. I encouraged my husband to lie on his side when he took his naps because at night, he slept on his back.

Pay particular attention to your loved ones feet, including the heels and toes. If you see areas of redness, place padding around that area, so it's not irritated further. I used many pillows and soft towels when putting Dean to bed. His feet and knees were placed on a big pillow. His arms were supported on rolled towels. If skin wounds are allowed to break open, it can take months to heal. As they say, an ounce of prevention is worth a pound of cure. In this case, it could not be more true.

Because foot care is so important, I recommend that you see a foot doctor to care for the toenails. A podiatrist can educate you in safe foot care.

Prevent Skin Injuries

One of the easiest, yet very important ways to keep skin healthy is with good hygiene. Your loved one's feet and legs need to be washed daily. This is also a good time to inspect the skin for tiny abrasions. Showers are best, but may not always be easy to do when balance problems make transferring into the shower unsafe. If a shower is not a daily option, a bed bath for all parts of the body is important. Changing soiled bed clothes and sheets helps keep skin healthy. Skin that is in constant contact with the toxic acids of old perspiration can become irritated.

Wearing shoes is also important. Some foot coverage helps prevent a skin abrasion if your loved one bumps his toes on the furniture leg. Shoes should have rubber soles to help prevent slips.

Staying hydrated with many glasses of water helps the immune system and the skin. In the later stages, I needed to remind Dean to drink. He didn't seem to be aware that he was thirsty. I realized that he was more alert when he was hydrated, so I encouraged him to drink all day long.

This list is not inclusive of all the ways that the immune system needs to be supported. It is advantageous for the caregiver to be ever vigilant. Healthy skin and careful hygiene can prevent many serious problems that take time and, of course, cause discomfort.

Digestive System

What we eat is very important when trying to keep our bodies healthy. It is an extremely important area for caregivers to research. When we become responsible for everything that another person eats, it can be an advantage and a disadvantage. The responsibility to be sure that our loved ones get all the necessary nutrients every day is huge. Caregivers might benefit from reading a library book about nutrition, vitamins and minerals. This chapter will not deal with that. Books are available at the library.

Nausea and Constipation

What does need to be explained are the problems of nausea and constipation that are common with LBD. If the digestive system stops working properly, your loved one can be miserable. Dean suffered with digestive problems for months. His every thought on some days centered on whether he could have a bowel movement. The nausea and constipation problems caused him more physical pain than any other LBD symptom.

Shortly after Dean started taking the pills for the diagnosis of Parkinson's disease, he began to develop chronic indigestion. The longer he was on the pills, the worse the nausea became. At the worst, it was all day long. If he ate, he was nauseated. If he didn't eat, he was more nauseated.

Constipation was one of the causes of nausea for Dean. The digestive muscles became inefficient at pushing wastes through the colon. His doctors told Dean that if he had a bowel movement every few days, he should not worry. That might be appropriate advice for some people. In my husband's case, he became chronically constipated. Besides severe nausea, the constipation caused abdominal discomfort, discomfort with the movements, and anxiety about moving the bowels. Dean became obsessed with going to the bathroom. We learned to discuss the relationship between various medications and the possible effects of constipation and/ or nausea with the doctors. When possible, we chose drugs that had fewer problems with nausea and constipation.

We tried the natural remedies of fruit pastes, prunes, and phospho-soda as laxatives. We tried the over-the-counter fibers that contained psyllium and mixed them with water or juice. This mixture actually worked against him, making the situation worse. When he finally would have a bowel movement, the stools were as hard as concrete and very difficult to pass.

Fortunately, a digestive specialist recommended a fiber product that did work for him. If he took a dose of the new fiber every morning, he had normal BMs and no more nausea. What a huge difference that made in his life.

Our message is to persevere. Surely something is out there to get the bowels working more normally. Your spouse will think you are a miracle worker when you find the right product, because it will make him feel like life is worth living again.

"Good" and "Bad" Foods

We found several foods that seemed to help the digestive system. A multivitamin coupled with a better diet took the extra 35 pounds off after he retired. His energy came back. When he went through a time of swelling in his ankles, I added extra greens to his diet in a morning green drink. The powder I used was pulverized barley grass, broccoli, parsley, and other dark green vegetables. The swelling went away.

Some foods had negative effects on Dean's health: alcohol, chocolate and sugar were the worst. I kept a "Don't Take This" list. A half glass of Sangria on vacation caused loud agitated dreams and restless sleep most of the night. A binge on chocolate at Halloween created a chocolate hang-over the next day. The after effects of heavy desserts or two donuts could rob him of needed clear thinking and good balance reactions for several hours. He learned that he would feel healthier if he avoided alcohol and quit his occasional alcoholic drinks himself. Chocolate and sugar were more difficult to limit.

The Excretory System

Incontinence

Incontinence is a common problem for persons with LBD because of the neurological effects on the bladder. Incontinence is defined as the inability to prevent accidents for urine or stool. As a person becomes weaker and more immobile, the frequency of the bowel and bladder accidents can increase. We prevented urgent bathroom trips by scheduling bathroom breaks about every two hours during the day. Dean couldn't always move fast enough to get to the bathroom after he had the urge to go. It worked very well.

Whether the accidents are due to the inability to move quickly or because of neurological problems, wearing a protective pad can provide tremendous assurance. The products are significantly more comfortable and dependable now than they were ten years ago. There are disposable briefs now on the market that don't even "crinkle" when a person walks.

Dealing with incontinence at night is a more complicated problem. When it was no longer safe for Dean to get up by himself, I had to get up to help him. He might call six times a night. The next day, both of us would feel like our brains were wrapped in cotton.

Our solution was voluntary incontinence. We used pads and mattress covers similar to what he used when he was in the hospital for the three-night-stay. I needed to try several different brands of adult diapers and extra pads until I found products that would keep the bed dry all night. His sleep improved substantially when he stopped getting out of bed 6-7 times a night to go to the bathroom. His shoulders stopped hurting. And I managed to get 7-8 hours of quality sleep most nights.

When dealing with incontinence, it is important to maintain hygienic conditions. The person will need to be cleaned with good wipes frequently when the soiled padded briefs are changed, just as a baby needs to be cleaned during each diaper change. Preventing skin irritations takes much less effort than tending to chafed skin later.

To be proactive, I used a waterproof pad on his lounge chair. The nice thing about caregiving for this generation is the variety of disposable products. When I found supplies I liked, I asked my local pharmacy to stock them for me.

The Skeletal System

Muscle and Tendon Injuries

Dean had many sprains and strains of muscles and tendons during his years with LBD. This was logical. As his strength and flexibility decreased, soft tissue injuries occurred. Dean would complain of a back twinge just by rolling over in bed.

During our active years playing tennis, we both used health and wellness magnetic pads and sleep products from a Japanese company.[25] (Disclaimer: these products would not have been used on Dean if he had any type of a pacemaker or stimulator that was regulated with magnetics.) The products seemed to lessen Dean's shoulder aches which allowed him to move more easily in bed. They allowed me to give him some comfort on any sore muscle area without putting another chemical product into his body.

It did help for him to do a regular stretching and strengthening program several times a week to keep his muscles as flexible as possible. If stretching becomes too difficult to do by himself, it might be worth having regular visits from a PT to assist the stretching exercises.

Injuries from Falls

We were lucky that he only dislocated the collar bone with a fall. He sustained many bruises but no broken bones. Caregivers might review Chapter 6 for important information to avoid falls.

Central Nervous System

Sleep Issues

Besides the expected neurological dysfunctions mentioned in the other chapters, Dean had another central nervous system problem that had to be remedied: insomnia. His abnormal sleep patterns were a big problem. We worked hard to figure out all the reasons that he was either sleeping too little, too much, or at the wrong times.

At one phase of the disease, he went through months with his days and nights mixed up. He would wake at 3:00 a.m. and not be able to go back to sleep. This would create a problem the next day when he couldn't stay awake. I found if I took him out of the house, he would be more apt to stay awake during the day. After a short nap in the morning, we would go somewhere. As long as we kept the naps to a reasonable amount of time, he still slept well at night. A snack before bedtime also helped to keep him asleep all night. Alcohol, heavy sugars, and antihistamine drugs could all create abnormal sleep patterns for him.

Dean's LBD played havoc with the need for sleep. As the disease progressed, he needed more and more sleep and fatigued more quickly after a nap. During the last year, anxiety produced a very fragile ability to stay asleep. He needed to call me several times a night. Sometimes, I would go to his room, and he would be calling me in his sleep. To allow me to get some sleep, we used a drug recommended by his doctor that allowed him to get a solid night of sleep. Amazingly, he woke alert and coherent in the morning. We had some of our best breakfast talks after nights on that pill.

Dream states can affect quality of sleep. Dean often had very animated dreams during the middle years of the disease. He would act out his dreams verbally and physically while he slept. I sometimes would enter his bedroom and watch him. He could look like he was fighting a war. Arm and legs were moving as fast as he could move them. He would shout directions to his dream partners. If he was having a dream that brought him laughter and happiness, I let him continue to sleep. If he was waging battle, I woke him in hopes the next section of the night might be less physically taxing.

Any stress, pain, or infection would result in a need for more sleep. After the shoulder injury, he slept for almost three days. Problems with any part of the body could trigger a need for more sleep. Any small or large problem wore him out physically and mentally and demanded more sleep.

At times I felt like the entertainer who spins plates. Any body system at any time could start to wobble and need concerted energy to get that body part back to good form. It was a hectic act to keep all his parts working on any given day. But when we could, he was generally able to display his normal witty personality. That was worth the effort.

Drugs in General Need to Be Discussed.

The primary treatment for maintaining function is an individually prescribed regimen of medicines. Many drugs are now available to help with the physical and mental aspects of LBD.

There are different drugs which target different functions of the brain. Some drugs do not react well with other drugs. This is not a good place to name names because so many options are available and so many different reactions can occur. What might not have worked for Dean might be a miracle drug for someone else.

I cannot emphasize strongly enough the importance of choosing a doctor who is current on what medications can and cannot do for your spouse. It is extremely important for the doctor to share openly with all family and caregivers which drugs to take and why; as well as which drugs not to take and why. As an example, our family doctor was very conscientious about checking on his computer for any potential drug reactions if a new drug was being considered.

He tried to be ever diligent to prevent using drugs that might have serious side effects. As careful as all our doctors were, Dean still received various medications that caused more harm than good. I would recommend that if two doctors are regularly following your spouse, i.e. a family practice doctor and a neurologist, they communicate with each other about changes in prescriptions. In our situation, I was the messenger delivering updates from one doctor to another. As conscientious as I was, we still had drug mishaps.

Drugs Known to Cause Problems for Many People with LBD

There are only two types of drugs that I feel need to be mentioned in this book. Forewarned is forearmed. The side effects of these particular types of drugs can be devastating.

Anticholinergic: The first type of drug contains anticholinergic ingredients.[26] Anticholinergic means that the chemicals in the product cause the drug to inhibit the affects of the neurotransmitter acetylcholine. Acetylcholine is a normal chemical that the body makes to help with brain functions such as memory, thinking, problem solving, as well as assisting with involuntary muscles, and stress reactions in the body. With a drug that is anticholinergic, healthy people may experience drying properties: less sinus drainage and perspiration. This is a common desired response for people who take antihistamines for colds and sinus drainage. Most urinary drugs are anticholinergic to help decrease leakage and frequent urination at night. Enough people with PD and LBD have negative reactions to products with anticholinergic properties that caregivers should be skeptical if any new drug ordered is considered anticholinergic. If a notebook is kept of products that cause negative reactions, patterns might begin to surface. This is a good topic to discuss with the doctors.

Dean had a violent reaction to one pill with anticholinergic properties. I came into his bedroom after his nap to find him extremely agitated. He didn't know who I was although he seemed to trust me. He wanted me to call the government and stop the conspiracy that was occurring. Bad people were trying to take over; and he wanted me to fight them off.

These manifestations were so severe that I had to admit him to the hospital. He was dehydrated, with a urinary tract infection and a sinus infection, in addition to a very bad reaction to the new medication. He was an inpatient for three days with only minimal recovery. The discharge home was the discharge from Hell. He was still out of his mind, flailing his arms, and unable to stand. It took three of us to get him into the house and into his bed. Most wives would have elected the discharge to an extended care facility. I knew if I could get him home, I had the skills to handle the situation until he could rebound.

He needed a hospital bed, restraints, and round the clock supervision for the next few days. It took six weeks to get him back to a healthy functioning state. Fortunately, we had a happy ending. He did recover from this drug episode in time to go on a cruise with close friends.

This is an example of what can happen if a person has a reaction to a particular type of drug. Some people need anticholinergic medications and do well. They might have problems with a different kind of medication. Caregivers will do well to monitor big changes after taking a new product or medication. I learned to check on-line for products that were anticholinergic. Surprisingly, I found that several products in my house were listed. They all went onto my "do not take" list.

The second warning applies to drugs that are considered antipsychotic drugs.[14] These drugs are frequently used to calm down people; however, they can have an adverse reaction in persons with LBD. Some antipsychotic drugs can also make the parkinsonism worse if they are dopamine blockers. Seroquel (quetiapine) and Clozaril (clozpaine) are antipsychotics that are usually safe to take in LBD, and may in fact be needed to help with the hallucinations, which can be severe in LBD patients. It is best to remember that all drugs are chemicals that are foreign to the body.

Sudden Adverse Reactions

One other important thing to remember is that any drug that worked well when your spouse was healthy may work differently after LBD. As an example of this, I will share our erectile dysfunction pill experience on a vacation. Believe the warning that low blood pressure can occur. After one E.D. pill and a big meal, Dean had a very strange reaction in a restaurant in New Orleans. When I came back from the restroom, he was immobile, rigidly sitting in the chair, with his eyes wide open, blank stare, and no blinking. It was as if he was asleep sitting up with his eyes open – except that I couldn't rouse him. I was about to call the emergency medical specialist's when he began to take sips of water that I offered to him through a straw. His pulse was normal, and his color was good so I continued to feed him sips of water until he finally turned his head and said, "What's up?" He didn't remember anything that happened. When I related this episode to our doctor at the next visit, his recommendation was to stop the erectile dysfunction drugs. They were too dangerous for Dean to use.

In Summary

Consider the following strategies to avoid drug reactions.

1. Take good notes on any effects of a particular food or drug. Report any incidents to the doctors. The medication might need to be stopped or possibly the dosage adjusted.

2. Drug effectiveness needs to be constantly checked. What worked at one point might not be effective later in the disease.

3. Most drugs have side effects. Some side effects were worse for quality of life and safety than the symptom the drug was prescribed to treat. Good communication with the doctors helped us determine how to get the best results with the least side effects from a minimum number of prescriptions.

Chapter 11

Understanding the Challenges of Declining Mental and Cognitive Abilities

God made everything beautiful in itself and in its time—but he's left us in the dark, so we can never know what God is up to, whether he's coming or going. I've decided that there's nothing better to do than go ahead and have a good time and get the most we can out of life. That's it—eat, drink and make the most of your job. It's God's gift.
—Ecclesiastes 3:11-13 The Message

Lewy Body Dementia is the second most common form of dementia after Alzheimer's disease.[27] In Chapter 2, I described the similarities and differences between Lewy Body Dementia, Parkinson's disease and Alzheimer's disease.

To help caregivers better understand the extent that the mental decline had on daily function, several have been described in this chapter. The decrease in mental processing is one of the main characteristics of LBD. It was one of the worse aspects for us to deal with. As Dean progressed in symptoms his thinking abilities could resemble those of a three-year-old child. He couldn't do math tasks and needed to be watched for safety issues. During the last 12 months, he occasionally functioned both mentally and physically like an 18-month-old child. Near the end of his life, there were days or parts of days that his balance and processing could be more like a 9-month-old child.

It is very difficult to make accommodations, if you can't appreciate what changes the disease process is producing. In patients I have worked with in my work facilities, family members have become very angry with the person struggling with LBD. When the family does not understand that functional capabilities come and go, wax and wane, they become angry if performance is radically different one day from the next. It certainly is not a logical pattern of deterioration.

It is even more frustrating when a loved one seems to be able to perform well for the doctor, visiting friends, or visiting children. These are called showtimes[14] and not a characteristic in other dementias such as AD.

It may help to understand that thinking abilities do not usually deteriorate overnight. It is a gradual process of symptoms. The LBD thinking vacillations (here and gone, here and gone) were a positive and a negative for me. I had to be careful not to get angry when Dean truly couldn't carry out a simple task. On the other hand, I was forever thankful for the periods of clear thinking that he did have during any particular day. I was thankful for his ability to show off with appropriate manners and conversations when we had guests or when family came to visit. I could get very frustrated with him the next day when he needed to sleep all day or was overly confused.

Fortunately for us, Dean had frequent periods when he was coherent with a sense of humor up to the day that he entered into a coma. I credit his ability to be coherent up to the end as the result of all the physical and mental exercises that we did together. A research project would be required to prove or disprove my theory, but I can hope that what we did helped. It is one of the reasons I wrote the book.

If the strategies and accommodations presented in this chapter can help other patients maintain some mental clarity, our book will be worthwhile. Losing one's mind is a terrible thing.

Our Experience With Dementia

Inability to Process Language

At times I would say something to my husband, and he wouldn't respond. He would need to ponder my words before he could reply. That lag time is not unusual in a brain dysfunction disease. On his worst days, he thought I was speaking another language because my words made no sense to him.

Understanding the meaning of my words was very important. One day when he was struggling to understand my directions for him to turn before sitting, he was able to tell me that he was having difficulty understanding my request. "I don't know what you mean when you tell me to TURN around before I sit on the bed." If I had not been trained to understand problems with cognition, I might have thought Dean was being silly or worse—sarcastic.

When your loved one has difficulty understanding your requests, try any or all of theses suggestions.

Use more than one type of communication method to get big ideas to stick. Early in the disease process, I had to repeat myself less often when I wrote in a calendar or had Dean write the events of the day or week into his calendar by his place at the table. Seeing and writing helped the hearing sense get new information to stick in the memory section of the brain. This is similar to writing spelling words five times as homework.

Talk in a normal tone, with normal volume. Do not yell. Yelling triggers anxiety and stress which shuts down all learning and processing. The words we use and how we say them can calm or agitate, even when our intentions are good and kind. Diana Waugh, RN, explains this very well in her book: I Was Thinking.[28]

Talk slower and use shorter sentences. Ask one idea, very simple questions or give very simple directions, such as, "Lunch time." Wait for a response. "Would you like soup today?" Wait. "Would you like salad today?"

Decrease talking when walking. Use hand gestures or touch to indicate direction.

Hallucinations

Hallucinations are seeing or perceiving that which is not there[17]. The presence of hallucinations is a characteristic of mental dysfunction. Newer drugs may be helpful. This is not a symptom to be ignored. If the hallucinations can be managed, quality of life may remain good. If they become severe, causing paranoia, the person will need to be in a facility equipped to deal with stronger medications for the irrational behaviors that are a result of the excessive fears.

Dean's drifted into a stage when the "nothingness" seemed to be very real. Two years after being diagnosed with Parkinson disease because of physical symptoms, my husband started to complain of many weird visions throughout the day. Every morning, Dean would regale me with stories of his night with his visitors: specters on the walls, aliens on his bed, or strange critters sleeping with him. He would call me many times during the day to show me what was in the room with him. At times I could understand his confusion. A curtain might be blowing with the breeze through the open window; or a shoe might be sticking out from under a chair. If I had something to show him, he did better than when I had no evidence to explain away the manifestation. Initially, I could teasingly joke about the aliens. Later, he became obstreperous and demanded that there were rodents such as mice and rats in our house. The severity of the visions was beginning to make him fearful, and our relationship contentious.

We were fortunate that our doctor was forthright with Dean. When Dean argued that the images could be real because no one had verified that they weren't really there, our doctor forcefully stated that they were not real, and he needed to stop persisting that they were. The doctor explained that to persist in believing in their existence could lead to the feeling that the little men and the armies were out to do him harm. With that escalation, life could become unbearable. Dean was shocked that our doctor was so forceful with him, but later worked very hard to keep the hallucinations in perspective. He would tell me what he saw, and we would laugh about the weirdo's maneuvering around in his mind.

We were also fortunate that new medications were approved for the mental aspects of LBD. When Dean added an anxiety pill to his daily routine, the hallucinations decreased. After he began a dementia medication, they decreased further.

Problem Solving

Most of us take our ability to solve problems for granted. It affects every action of every day. The simple tasks of choosing which clothes to wear, tying the shoes, or turning on the stove to boil water are easy problem solving tasks that disintegrate with LBD. The more technical skills that most people consider as problem solving are computing a math problem, sending an email, or balancing the check book. All of these more complicated skills were wiped out for my husband before anyone suspected that he was becoming unhealthy.

The second examples above require a working memory bank in the brain. Math facts, once learned, are stored. When needed, we "think" and the facts pop into our minds. To do email on the computer, a sequence of decisions must be made. We need to remember how to turn the computer on, which icon stands for the email program, and how to do all the steps to write and send the message. When a disease has either robbed our brain bank of our stored memories or destroyed our abilities to get to the brain bank to pull out information, we can't solve problems.

Dean referred to his thinking ability as being foggy brained. As we can't see anything around us when we are driving in a fog, Dean felt he couldn't think clearly. It might be easier to understand the difficulties with problem solving if we realize that on foggy brain days, people with LBD live only in the present. If a problem occurs, only solutions immediately present will be used. When Dean could not get the right buttons to work to tilt his power reclining chair to upright, he might begin to use crazy body contortions to get out of the chair over the elevated foot rest. It did no good to give him pictures to demonstrate which buttons did which actions. It did no good to place an alerting bell near his chair that would have called me for help. What he could see immediately in front of him was his reality. He needed to get out of the chair, so he attempted to climb over all barriers. I learned to recognize any strange sound from anywhere in the house.

Any financial information was difficult for Dean to hold on to. Early in the disease process, when the financial planner suggested strategies, Dean would nod his head and agree. It did not stay. The next day he would not remember any of the discussion. Because he realized that he could not process complicated matters anymore, we had Power of Attorney documents drawn up by our lawyer for medical directives and financial decisions.

Part of the problem solving difficulty was his loss of sequencing abilities. He could not put tasks in order. When explaining something to him that would happen in the future, I was more successful if I related the whole story, and then broke it down into one-step directions until he got it: "I am leaving for church while you are napping. Eric will be here to take you to church. I will meet you at church. Eric will then go home." If he could put it into his own words with the right ideas, I knew he had it.

Memory Loss

Five years before we had a diagnosis of LBD, Dean was not able to remember work he had done the day before. He carried notebooks in his shirt pocket to remind himself what he needed to do next. It didn't get better after he retired.

How we played games will describe the adjustments we made throughout the disease process. He could play gin rummy and Chess™ in

2006 and beat me, but he could not do math computations or remember how to get onto the computer. When those games became too difficult we enjoyed crossword puzzles that we could do together, and Chinese Checkers™ with pegs. When he no longer could focus on the pegs or small print, we played thinking games like Cranium™ and Trivial Pursuit™. We tried to answer the questions as a team. In the last year, he was only able to enjoy our granddaughters color games and a simple dice game, but I needed to keep track of the score.

Living primarily in the present moment affected Dean's ability to complete tasks. Sporadically throughout the day memory would be very short. Dean could take his pills, and a few minutes later reach for the pill tray to take more pills. I could remind him to put on his shoes so that we could leave the house. If I did not stay right by his side, he might lie down on the bed and be asleep instead of putting the shoes on. On the positive side, Dean's favorite TV program, NCIS was always fresh and entertaining no matter how often we watched a particular rerun.

As a caregiver of someone with Alzheimer's and LBD, you should expect your spouse's memory of events, places, and people to decline. Dean's memory definitely declined, but fortunately, with the fluctuations, never fully left him. He always knew me and our family members and occasionally, he would amaze me by remembering something that I had forgotten; even into the last stage of this disease. When we were stuck in Nashville during the flood (six months before he passed) he reminded me that we had a doctor's appointment that I would need to cancel. Amazing!

Wandering

When Dean was in one of his periods of foggy thinking, he would wander aimlessly through the house. Sometimes he could tell me what he was wandering to get; and other times, he would forget before he could get to his target. Most of my husband's walking was purposeful. He would walk to get a drink, go to the bathroom, or shift to a more comfortable chair. If he couldn't tell me why he was up, I watched closely to try to determine what was going through his mind.

When wandering is happening, it is important to monitor all actions. I would find items in strange places, such as a pot holder in the refrigerator, a container of ice cream on the stove, and worst of all, the TV remote control far from the TV. Because Dean couldn't think back in his mind to recall where he might have put the remote, I could spend an hour searching the entire house trying to find our precious remote control. It was as valuable as gold. And to think, my parents always had to get up to change channels.

Of real concern were the wanderings at night. One night Dean separated his shoulder during a fall at 4:00 A.M. behind a closed and locked door. Once I jimmied the lock, got into the room, got him up off the floor and made his shoulder comfortable, I could see that the room was a mess. He had been rifling through drawers, and tugging at clothes in the closet. Everything was out of place.

Fearing for his safety and the safety of the house, I secured Swiss cow bells to the inside of the bedroom door, then weighted the door open with a cast iron door stopper. When Dean got out of bed by himself and tried to close the door, I heard the bells immediately. That worked for a long time.

Strategies to Stimulate Mental Processing

I truly understand that the deterioration of the mental processing can be very challenging and emotionally draining. It was the worst thing I had to deal with. During those times when Dean's memory became very short, I needed to understand yet again that this was real. He was giving me the best he had to give. If he could remember, he would remember. If he could move faster, he would move faster. No amount of criticism or fussing at him would get him to complete any task any quicker. Fussing would just make him sad. In fact, he really couldn't understand what he had done to get me fussing. He was not able to change, so I had to. Instead of fussing at his inabilities, I developed various strategies that seemed to help us both minimize the stresses created by his dementia.

Gentle Reminders Can Help

I finally learned to stop saying, "I told you about that!" I was more helpful if I would review names and particulars for all the people he would be seeing before we entered a room with many friends. He seemed to enjoy his conversations with friends if I was not directly by his side. He could tell his *stories*, and I wouldn't be there to correct the details. The family could get him very involved in conversations if we picked subjects that he was passionate about in his youth. Those memories stayed with him the longest.

There is a time to cry and another to laugh…
—Ecclesiastes 3:4 The Message

Humor

Humor helps strengthen thinking as lifting weights strengthens muscles. It takes intelligence and sharp recall to make the analogy between one idea and another. Dr. Carla Hannaford, writes extensively in her book, <u>Awakening the Child Heart</u>, how stress imposed on a child becomes a destructive element and actually impedes learning in the classroom[29]. In LBD, the goal for the caregiver is to use all activities possible to activate the thinking part of the brain. Humor doesn't cost anything and it is a wonderful tonic for the ongoing stresses during the day. Nothing works better than a hardy laugh to break down a heavy load of stress.

Dean maintained some wittiness throughout all stages of the LBD and remained able to laugh at himself. The disease gave us great material to turn into a good laugh. During one of our neighborhood walks on a beautiful summer day when he was using a rolling walker, Dean calmly mentioned that he was losing his pants. The pants looked okay to me so I pooh-poohed the possibility. He very calmly responded with, "I AM losing my pants! In fact I just dropped my shorts in the middle of the neighborhood." I looked at his ankles and, sure enough, there was his favorite orange shorts lying on the ground. As I reached down to help pull up the shorts, I saw our neighbors across the street smiling and waving with enjoyment. We both began laughing so hard, I had trouble holding up the pants and getting him into the house.

Dean used wit to try to understand his body changes. During our first doctor visit in 2005, he described his walking difficulty as "stumble-itis" and his focusing problems as "foggy thinking".

In the later years, when he definitely was dealing with loss of both physical and mental skills on a daily basis, we sought out humor as a quest. I read him all of the Stephanie Plum, bounty hunter books by Janet Evanovich.[18] Every morning, I read two chapters. At times we both would be laughing hysterically. I would need to stop to wipe tears before I could continue reading. Our reading sessions created wonderful memories for the two of us.

Reading the books to Dean had great benefits besides the laughter. He thought about the material and processed the humor — good thinking exercises. He also anchored the information and was able to retell some funny parts to friends. This was an exercise in strengthening Dean's short term memory.

Dean maintained the ability to tease and kibitz with his buddies and my brother even on the day before going into a coma. I only have one in-depth 'case' of LBD, but I feel the power of humor was one force that helped my husband keep his mental faculties up to the end, and helped me stay focused.

Decrease Anxiety

When Dean became anxious, the logical thinking part of his brain would shut down. We learned that he did worse if I tried to hurry him. If I planned ahead, his ability to focus on the activity would be maximized. I learned to tell Dean that our time to leave was at least 15 minutes earlier than it really was, because it took about 30 extra minutes to get out of the door for an outing.

Adjust the Schedule

He could become immersed in a task. The very act of brushing his teeth and rinsing with mouthwash could take 15 minutes when it only took five in the healthy years. I would occasionally just stand and watch. Dean seemed to ponder as he gathered the supplies: toothbrush, "check", paste, "check", water, "check". Next, he might blow his nose or comb his hair. He would proceed with the brushing, and do it very thoroughly. He might rinse three times and then repeat the brushing.

It could take a full minute to get the top off of the bottle of mouthwash. He would thoroughly put all supplies back, and wipe his hands and mouth; then comb his hair again. He might get fully out of the bathroom before turning around to use the mouthwash again. His efforts needed to be appreciated and every minute valued because he felt he had done what he set out to do and did a very satisfying job. So, I adjusted by scheduling in the extra time, and busied myself with other tasks while I waited.

Maintain Familiar Surroundings To Decrease Stress

We found out how drastically a lack of familiarity can affect the mental status of a person with dementia when Dean was admitted to the hospital for an infection and drug reaction. He was admitted because he was not coherent, could not stand, and was experiencing violent hallucinations. Even though the drug was out of his system after two days in the hospital, his mind was not clearing. In fact, he was becoming more confused and hostile. Our doctor explained that the unfamiliarity of the surroundings and the fact that I was not there to reassure him 24 hours a day was creating more problems. A few days after he returned home, he began to think and act more normally.

I was concerned that he would become anxious anytime I was away from the house, but he was fine as long as he was with familiar people who made the effort to reassure him. My son used a baby monitor in Dean's room for a four-night visit when I needed to be away. Dean barely had to whisper and Todd would be up to reassure him. The monitor worked so well, I purchased one to use at our house.

Dean would be calmer on nights when he had a night light. We learned to take one with us when we were traveling. Understanding his limitations and insecurities helped us avoid those situations where he could be confused by his environment and feel abandoned and alone.

We reduced stress by organizing supplies needed when leaving the house. Part of the problem with short-term memory loss was putting things away in a place where the items could be found later. I needed to know where his shoes, wallet, and keys were. Dean could not walk back through the tasks of the past day or week to think where he might have left keys. If we had to search all the pants pockets for his house key, it could take an extra 30 minutes and I would become frustrated and grumpy. I organized the task of leaving the house by giving him a fanny pack that contained extra pills, key, wallet, glasses, and handkerchief. The pouch was always left by the cane he used for outings. We then had needed items readily waiting. This simple change greatly allowed us to get out the door quickly and calmly.

I adopted a "What you see is what you get" strategy. I wanted my kitchen counters clear and pretty, but that didn't work for Dean. He needed things in plain sight and always in the same place: pills by his plate, cereal box on the sink counter. Early on, I would lose my patience when he couldn't find some item that was in plain sight, right where I told him it would be. I may be a little slow in catching on, but I finally realized Dean was not calling for me, just to annoy me. He really couldn't find something that he thought he needed. The more in the open and in specific places that I put things, the less he needed to call me. Listed below are a few examples of what worked for us.

All dishes always in the same cupboard spots

Food was always stored in the same approximate place in the refrigerator

His jackets were always on the right of the closet, mine on the left.

Remote control was always by his favorite chair and marked with hot pink tape

Favorite clothes hung on pegs outside his closet door

It was worth the effort to keep him comfortable. When he wasn't stressed, I was happier. The planning and structuring in the home was extended to all areas of Dean's life: the car, restaurants, vacations and visits overnight with family.

Maintain a Familiar Schedule To Decrease Stress.

We followed a routine for the day and for the week as I had done when raising my children. I tried to arrange outings to fit around his nap times. He had specific channels on the TV for sports or news that he preferred. I kept the TV running even during his naps. If the TV was turned off, it posed a problem for him to get back to his favorite channels.

I made a list of his daily activities and posted it on the refrigerator. If I had a friend or family member staying with Dean for the day, all his needs were spelled out in detail. Each month, I needed to revise the list to reflect changes, i.e. two naps a day instead of one.

Set Goals to Exercise Memory

Having a purpose encourages a person to think long term. This is tremendously important. It is easy to give up if all expectations are stripped from the options list. As a PT and later as a caregiver, I heard these comments from other families: "I can't play golf anymore because I can't lift the bag in and out of the car." "I can't eat in public anymore because I occasionally spill something." "I can't get out of the house because I need a wheelchair and I have steps." "I would rather stay home just in case I might have a dribbling accident." In all these examples, a small manageable barrier became a major obstacle. When hope leaves, it takes purpose with it.

The first step in setting a goal is to determine the desired outcome. What would your spouse still like to do to fill his days? What prevents him from doing that? Is there any way that modifications could make it happen? What is plan B?

Big goals become reality by mastering a series of small manageable steps. It is during the small steps that modifications can be introduced. Modifications can be small or large. A small modification might be trying the adult diaper system to prevent the problems with dribbling when the person leaves the house. A large modification would be contracting to have a ramp built over the steps leading into the house. When caregivers share big dreams, modifications can happen to allow the big dreams to become reality.

Setting goals was possibly one of the best activities to keep both Dean's mind sharp and body fit. Planning for a vacation was a pleasant normal activity to do together. We both had a reason to get out of bed each morning. We had exercises to do, walks to take, brochures to read, activities to plan for our next trip.

Activate the Adventure Attitude

Each family reading this can only do the best they can. Our message is not the size of the adventure, it is acquiring an adventure mentality for both the caregiver and the spouse. With a little extra planning, great memories can be made with trips to the doctor's office. Our message is to have fun doing whatever you are doing for two reasons: the joy when you experience it the first time, and the pleasure of telling the story later.

In fact it is the really goofy, unique LBD scenarios like these two stories that I remember with the most pleasure.

The Seven Hour Overnight Flight to Spain

I logically concluded that if I could get Dean through the ordeal of an overnight flight, I could manage the cruise for a week. I took an inflatable neck pillow for him, hoping that it would hold his head in place while he slept on the plane. Between 3 and 4 a.m., he was trying to unwind and sleep, but as soon as he drifted off, he would begin to have relaxed erratic arm and leg movements. These are perfectly fine in his spacious queen-sized bed at home. It didn't work well in a confined airplane seat. Every time his arm stretched out, he hit the seat in front of him and woke up. This was a test for me. I was prepared to put him right back on a plane and take him home if he was a physical and mental mess when we got to Spain.

I deduced that if I could cradle him in my arms and hold his arms down, he might be able to stay asleep. If he got some sleep, he would not be so overly tired the next morning. I actually raised the arm rest between us, turned sideways in my seat, and wormed one of my legs between Dean and his seat back. I wrapped my other leg over his legs to keep them steady and pulled him into my arms with his head on my shoulder. It was a good idea but not a good plan. Besides being very uncomfortable for me, my legs stuck out into the aisle.

With further shifting and wiggling, I managed to sit with my legs forward in a way that I could pull him into my arms. I wrapped my arms around him, restrained his arms and supported his head on my shoulder. He slept like a baby for the last two hours of the flight to Barcelona. But in that position, I did not get any sleep all night. Dean did very well when we landed and loved the city tour later in the day. I loved the nap I took slumped in the back of the van during the city tour.

Dean's Adventure When Alone on the Cruise

My second story revolves around the modifications we made for the day that I was to see the Vatican in Rome while Dean was to spend the day on the ship. He was thrilled that he was staying back by himself, allowing me to see something that I dearly wanted to see. I was apprehensive about leaving him, but he assured me that he would be fine.

For two days, he practiced learning how to get to the small restaurant just to the left of our cabin. I put a sign on the inside of our door that had an arrow pointing to the left so he would be headed in the correct direction. I made him a map and put it in a plastic nametag holder to wear around his neck. I told the cabin staff what was happening in case they found him lost in another hallway. He had books, a TV, and his bed for naps. I gave him a kiss, said a little prayer, and left.

When I came into the cabin eight hours later, Dean was lying on his bed with the cabin phone in his hand. He looked bedraggled and fully confused. I asked him who he was calling. He said, "You! I want you to come home!" He had ventured out and had walked around many areas of the ship. He did find the restaurant. He did get lost. He did re-find the cabin, and he was exhausted! It was not easy for me to leave him; and it was not easy for him to stay in unfamiliar surroundings by himself, but we both did it. I appreciated his great effort to let me go on that excursion, and he developed a new appreciation for how much he relied on me.

In Summary

Challenging a spouse to stay mentally active can be worthwhile. Using humor and more time to do daily tasks can decrease anxiety. Making adjustments to assure familiarity with routines may help a spouse stay productive. And finally, setting goals that you both need to work hard to achieve, may not only keep him thinking normally, it may provide a basket of memories that you can store in your heart forever.

Chapter 12

Mannerisms Seen on a Poor Functioning Day

a time to break down,
—Ecclesiastes 3:3 RSV

The course of Dean's disease was like a roller coaster ride. I never knew what to expect in the morning. He could be fully alert and talking about politics, or describing the little aliens that sat on the end of his bed all night. During the high moments, my husband of 39 years was in the room with me. No one would suspect that he had a disease. He acted like any other older gentleman. Even during his last hospital stay, on the afternoon before he went into a coma, he was fully alert and talking appropriately about football teams with my brother.

As the LBD became more intense, the normal personality showed up fewer mornings or lasted only till about 10:00 A.M. Mannerisms on those poor functioning days could be extremely challenging for me to understand. Those were the low points. As hard as he tried, all circuits were not firing in his thinking brain. In this chapter, I have described several of the weird mannerisms that Dean exhibited in hopes that these descriptions may offer some understanding for other caregivers if their loved one happens to board this same roller coaster.

Initially, Dean was strong and healthy physically, but he was thinking about things as if he was on a different planet. I have used terms that are Judy-isms. They may not have the same definition elsewhere. Dean seemed to catch onto and respond to these terms. At least I was able to get his attention for a short while.

Futzing is a term I used to describe time wasted on frivolities.

On these mornings when he was not mentally on target, I had to watch every action he did. He would fuss with anything he could get his hands on for no apparent reason. Anything might go into his mouth: plastic ties or nuts and bolts. He unscrewed the pepper shaker one day as if it was something he had never seen before. It would make some difference if I would say "quit futzing", but didn't stop him for long. I could divert him if I placed a good snack at his table mat: raisins, peanuts, almonds, or walnuts. He would munch and stay out of trouble. When he began to choke on his food, I needed to find a safer snack.

Gibberish was talking, but making no sense.

At times the words were not English. A few times, the coordination for his tongue was so poor, that he acted as if he was drunk. On those days, when he tried to talk, all the words ran together and his speech sounded garbled. I learned to immediately check his blood pressure to see if it was too high or too low. Both conditions could affect this talking ability and would require an appropriate pill.

The first time this happened, I called our family doctor because I was afraid Dean had had a stroke. He suggested I give him sips of water, check his blood pressure, and let him take a nap. He didn't seem surprised. For good reason, when Dean woke up, he was fine.

The inability to stop an action could be a problem.

When pouring cereal or milk, he just kept pouring. It gave new meaning to the term, "My cup runneth over."[30] It was sort of funny to see his pancakes swimming in a pool of syrup one day in a restaurant. He loved them.

I never got used to these idiosyncrasies. Maybe if he always did this, I could have adjusted. It was sporadic and always caught me by surprise. These next weird mannerisms were directly related to low points in the disease that affected both his mental and physical functioning.

Dropsie

I used the term dropsie to describe Dean's inability to sustain a muscular contraction while doing a task. The term made sense to him and is not related to the old medical condition referring to swelling in the arms or legs. It was such a dramatic happening when it occurred that we needed to have a label for it.

In an attempt to take a sip from a cup, the muscles that were lifting and holding the cup would quit, and his hands and the cup would fall into his lap. Occasionally the arms and hands would fly up into the air before they dropped to his lap. This was usually when he was trying to carry a bowl or plate filled with food. Cheerios would fly everywhere. Plastic dishes became the logical choice for Dean's dinnerware. Needless to say, this was messy and embarrassing. There was no warning for his sudden lack of coordination. He might exhibit his dropsie one day and then not again for a week.

It started in his hands much sooner than in his legs. Dean's knees would buckle without warning. Without my help, he would fall to the floor. One day, his knees buckled every time he tried to stand up. One would think if this happened one day, it would happen every day, but it didn't. The next day, he could walk again without the buckling.

We adjusted to the spilling problems in several ways. If I asked him if it was a dropsie day, he could usually tell me yes or no. We avoided the spills at pot luck dinners because I would carry both plates. At home, he stopped trying to help me clean up the table and didn't try to carry his plate to the sink.

Seizure-like Episodes:

These weird mannerisms were very scary; but the doctors explained that they were just a normal symptom of the LBD disease. If your loved one has something like this, it is best to notify his doctor to be sure that he is aware that these are occurring.

Dean would lose consciousness, sometimes for as long as 30 seconds. During this time his arms and legs would flail with random movements. We would need to ease him to the floor because he would have no balance, even while he was sitting in a chair. We would stay at this side until he came around and then we could get him back into chair where he would be fine.

These can be a serious concern. If your loved one slides out of the chair onto the floor while in this state, you may need to call for emergency help to get him up from the floor to a safe place. There did not seem to be any pattern to these seizure-like occurrences.

Closing Thoughts

Fortunately, LBD symptoms waxed and waned. Dean never dropped to the lows and stayed there. While waiting for him to bounce back up, I needed to adjust. I helped feed him, and held him tighter during the transfers from chair to bed because he was unsafe. We hoped the next day would be better. Other wives have reported to me that late in the disease, their husbands did not regain mental function and did not know who they were.

There were days during the last year when his thinking was too deficient to be able to make any decision. "What would you like for breakfast?" was too difficult for him to grasp. If watching a movie on TV, he couldn't follow the plot. If trying to put his shirt on, he might have it upside down.

During the last month, the periods of decreased mental alertness occurred several times a day. He might be alert for an hour after a nap with appropriate comments. I knew another nap was needed when he couldn't keep his eyes open, or started to talk incoherently again. The last month he was sleeping 12 hours at night from 7:30 p.m. till 7:30 a.m. He would be alert and happy until 9:00. He took naps from 9 -11, and 1-4:00. By 7:30 p.m. Dean was done for the day.

As the disease progresses, bizarre movements will happen. They may appear as described above; or they may look totally different. I would suggest securing help in the home when the mannerisms become so unconventional that you, the caregiver, do not know what to do to keep your loved one safe. A visiting nurse may be a good resource to help determine if any of these need further medical attention. Hospice assistance can always be called into the home with an incurable disease. Hospice can be started and even stopped if your loved one gets significantly better. These are late stage mannerisms and once started will continue to happen on an ongoing basis. If they become severe and frequent, it may be impossible to continue care for your loved one in the home setting.

Chapter 13

Potential Members of the Support Team

Lewy Body Dementia is an overwhelming disease. Caregivers will need help increasingly as the disease devastates normal mental and physical abilities. In this chapter, I have broken down the types of support that I found extremely valuable. We can't use help that we don't know exists.

Doctors

The doctors on your medical support team should be familiar with all the Parkinson's Plus diseases, of which LBD is just one. Some diseases may look like PD initially, but are in fact unique diseases with specific treatment options. The medical team should be set in place early in the disease process. This may include a primary care physician as well as neurology specialists. As other symptoms surfaced, such as digestion problems, I needed still other doctors. The marriage of both the large university-based clinic and the family doctor practice seemed to be the best fit for us.

Our university neurology group was very helpful with family education programs to explain the particulars of living with movement disorders. They hosted seminars featuring expert speakers on all aspects of a movement disease. I appreciated their knowledge on newest medications and research evidence.

Communication was very important to the specialists. I could reach our neurologist easily via an email system. He provided tremendous support to me throughout all stages of the disease by responding to me within 24 hours of an email request. My contact with other doctor groups required phone calls, long waits on hold, and requests submitted through voice messages. These did not get addressed nearly as quickly as the email system. I hope an email option becomes the choice with all doctors of patients requiring long term care.

The university doctors were linked to a vast number of adjunct specialists who provided in-depth evaluations for various symptoms. Some of these specialists were very helpful. Others made Dean feel like he was a pawn in a chess game. It further confused him.

Because the neurology group was not close to our town, Dean was also followed by our family practice group of doctors. When Dean required hospitalizations, I chose our local hospital. Our family doctors admitted him and treated him during those stays.

The primary advantage of maintaining contact with our family doctor was familiarity. This was especially important as the symptoms increased. Dean felt comfortable asking our family doctor difficult questions. When he told Dean to stop claiming that the hallucinations were real, it had an impact. Dean eventually was able to say, "My mind is playing tricks on me again."

On one visit, Dean asked his doctor how much time he could expect to live with this disease. This was an extremely difficult question for him to ask and reflects the high regard Dean had for his doctor friend. The answer was shocking. Dean expected to hear upwards of 20 years. When he heard 5-10 after the diagnosis, the news put him in a tailspin for a couple of days.

Dean could have quit or become reenergized. He became energized. Realizing that time was shorter than he had anticipated, he worked harder to remain healthy. I credit the positives in our last two years together as Dean's purposeful choice to make the time left to him meaningful.

For me, it was extremely important that I was appreciated by all the doctors on Dean's team. I needed to have doctors who would continue to listen to me and treat me as a valued team member. I needed my opinions to be respected. Doctors have knowledge and skills that are essential in the treatment process; but a spouse on the front line, fighting this battle 24/7, has vast knowledge and skills. I encourage a caregiving spouse to validate her/his worth and to expect a mutual respect from all members of the care team. Only someone observing daily habits can relate a change in those habits to the doctors.

Nurses

Visiting nurses assisting in the home can be a valuable addition to the medical team. After Dean's first hospitalization, our doctor recommended a visiting-nurse-visit once a week. She kept track of vital information: blood pressure, temperature, and heart function. She added a valuable perspective while monitoring Dean's vacillating health needs. A nurse visit may be extremely valuable for patients that have other related maladies in addition to the neurological complications. Our nurse suggested equipment that might make care easier. I appreciated the opportunity to sound out concerns once a week with a professional. If I had concerns as a trained medical professional, I can assume that non-medical caregivers would find the nurse visit equally valuable.

The Elder Services Program

The purpose of the program was to support families who want to care for loved ones in their own homes. These services were initiated after Dean returned home from the hospital. A care coordinator came to our home to do an intake evaluation, which was needed to determine if he qualified for services. Services are extensive and affordable. Besides the visiting nurse, Dean was eligible for an aide for bathing, light duty house work, and meal preparation. If a cost was attached to services, it was on a sliding scale dependent on monthly income minus expenses incurred for his care. Possible services provided by our county program were as follows:

Life-connect monitoring would have allowed Dean to call for help if he fell and was not near a phone. He merely had to push a button on a wrist bracelet. We subscribed to this program at a reduced rate.

Home maintenance projects that pertained to Dean's care were arranged by our contact person. We had a hand-held shower head installed in his shower.

"Meals on Wheels" was available to provide a light lunch and hot dinner meal five days a week.

Respite care was a feature allowing a patient to be cared for when a caregiver needed to be away from the home for a period of time. The contact coordinator could arrange a short stay in a care facility. If care would have become too difficult for me to continue in our home, our care coordinator would have helped me find a suitable nursing home where Dean could have lived.

Equipment purchases were facilitated. Our care coordinator suggested a rail for the bed and ordered it from a medical supply vendor for us. The cost was discounted.

Physical, Occupational, and Speech Therapy Services

Home therapy care can greatly assist caregiving. The positive changes in abilities can be dramatic with rehabilitation programs. Equipment can be suggested and ordered.

Physical therapy is needed to teach ambulation, equipment use, stair climbing, transfers, and bed mobility techniques to the family. A physical therapist can also provide excellent rehabilitation after any serious injury to bones or soft tissue. The PT should be able to teach how to move safely around the house and in and out of cars. If the caregiver is not able to provide stretching and strengthening exercise, the PT can administer an exercise program.

At times, when the disease was raging and Dean was going into a new phase, it was very helpful to be able to call my brother and sister-in-law, both trained physical therapists, for their perspective. My brother provided physical therapy assistance at various times during the five years. His work with Dean helped keep his shoulders working well. Without good arm strength to help with transfers, I might not have been able to keep Dean at home.

An occupational therapist teaches daily care, dressing, managing in a shower, transferring onto a commode, or using eating utensils. An OT will also be able to assist with equipment needs to ease care.

Either a PT or an OT can order equipment. Wheelchairs may need to be measured to fit the person. A hydraulic lift can be a tremendous help if standing transfers become unsafe. One small person can be trained to lift a very big man easily and safely out of bed to a wheelchair. The need for lifts must be evaluated by a therapist and ordered through medical equipment vendors.

A Speech and Language Pathologist may be required at some point to assess speech difficulties or choking problems. The SLP may also be able to offer strategies for the cognitive deficiencies.

You, as the caregiver, have the right to "interview" the agency responsible for contracting with you to provide allied care personnel in your home. The therapists who come into your home claiming to be therapists should be licensed physical therapists, physical therapy assistants, occupational therapists, or occupational therapy assistants. Speech and Language Pathologists or speech therapists also need to be licensed.

Care Personnel

I hired a few dependable people to come in to relieve me on specific days during the week. I could shop for groceries, do errands, or even work out with full knowledge that Dean was being well cared for by experienced caregivers. Agencies are staffed with caregivers who can provide these services when the family does not have a reserve of people qualified to help. It is good to have an agency in the wings when a neurological motor dysfunctional disease is diagnosed. It would mean one less search after a discharge from a hospital.

Confidants

Both of us needed to have other people in our lives to lean on for support. I trusted family and friends when they came in to help with his care.

I needed other women who had walked this walk before me. Their advice and counsel was valuable. When one friend told me that Dean had moved into the phase of the disease where he needed me home all day, I was shocked. I had not planned to quit my job for another year. As I saw his condition through her eyes, I realized that she was right. I did quit work and had a whole year with him that I would not have had if she had not been honest. Every caregiver needs companions on her support team who will be courageously honest.

Some friends just listened. My email buddies were always readily available and vitally important during the last year, when I couldn't leave Dean alone. They were my lifeline to the outside world. Sometimes I got funny cartoons, sometimes political information, sometimes mushy, syrupy-sweet messages about friendship. The message was not as important as the fact that I was on someone's mind.

Dean relied on me for all the medical decisions, but he needed other men to validate that he was more than some guy with a disease. I organized an evening-with-a-friend for several years. Each week, I scheduled a different buddy to come in and sit with him while I played tennis. Some talked politics, some played games with him, and others brought in funny videos. I always prepared snacks so they could have a good social visit. He really was energized by those guys. He could be foggy-brained with me all day, but alert and witty with his buddies.

Dean had a group of work friends that stayed true to him throughout the course of his disease. He was very motivated with these guys. It was amazing how he was able to click into his engineer persona when they were around. They always treated him as an intelligent, capable person; and he responded well to their affirmations. True friends are those who are willing to help carry your load.

Emotional Counselor

A pastor, priest, rabbi, or counselor should definitely be a part of the support team. I had two pastors whom I could schedule to see as I needed. I did a fairly good job of holding my emotions together, but there were times when I needed to quietly scream. Their sustaining insights helped give me the strength to persevere. More importantly, they never failed to compliment me on my choice to be a caregiver. It was vitally important for me to hear that.

In conjunction with the emotional support, I strongly suggest becoming affiliated with a house of worship. We did not join our church until Dean was already sick. We had been attending a mega church that was not in our home town. I realized that I needed a church close to home. The people in our new congregation welcomed us with open arms. The benefits are innumerable. We had a place to go for food and fun with people who were happy to see us. We had a weekly service that offered beautiful music and spiritual revitalization. This congregation provided a bank of people who provided home maintenance assistance. I had a ramp built, electrical work done, and consultations for a leaky roof. I found care personnel in the congregation who provided trusted care for Dean while I got away for an hour or two.

I didn't expect Dean to be able to make friends at that late compromised stage of his life. He did. Amazingly, many of the men in the congregation were able to see deep within the rubble caused by the disease. They gently searched below the layers to find the core of what made Dean a gentle giant. They saw a witty, well educated, generous, athletic, person who always treated others the way that he wished to be treated himself.

Developing a support team to deal with all the many aspects of a deteriorating disease is so very important. First-time caregivers will start their caregiving duties just as parents start their parenting: by throwing themselves into the "job". There is no rehearsal. We all learn as we go. Professionals and friends with experience can offer tremendous service to make the ordeal easier for everyone involved.

Chapter 14

Preparing for Financial Decisions

A time to plant, and another to reap,
—Ecclesiastes 3 The Message

Most caregivers in America are volunteers, family members who are willing to accept the duties of caring for a sick relative. More wives than husbands care for a spouse.[1] Unfortunately, as the disease intensifies, the caregiver must, not only face the stresses and emotional turmoil caused by the disease; they often assume the burden of dealing with the financial issues.

I was fortunate when dealing with the financial challenges. Dean insisted that I be involved with all money issues from the beginning of our marriage. I knew where all the accounts were, and approximately how much we had to live on if I worked or if I stayed home to care for him. What a priceless gift he gave to me.

Navigating through the financial maze can be more stressful than dealing with the disease. It doesn't need to be that way. Following are a few suggestions that can eliminate some of the financial hassles for the surviving spouse. Certainly these questions need to be answered as soon as either spouse learns that he or she has a serious illness, whether the disease is curable or not. Even more logical, these matters should be discussed before anyone becomes sick, when everyone is thinking calmly.

At the risk of offending, I am going to lie this on the discussion table. A disease is not affected by the choice to discuss financial issues and end of life decisions with a spouse. Specifically, making a will and discussing where the funds are will not hasten the end of life or make a disease worsen. Conversely, refusing to talk about financial matters will not prevent a disease from attacking our bodies or increasing in severity. Diseases don't know and don't care.

Become Informed About Finances

The people who will care are those who will be handling our finances after we are gone. Dean and I made our wills in our 30s and always talked about money together. If I wasn't smart enough to understand money, or sufficiently adept to take care of needs before Dean passed, I surely would have had to get smart and savvy quickly after he was gone. He didn't want me to be forced to get smart in a hurry.

All of this information is equally as important for an aging parent to share with the caregiving son or daughter.

Either spouse can pass first. I suggest that both know all about the finances.

Is there a will?	Where is it?
Is there a safe deposit box?	Where is the key?

If a financial planner is helping to manage finances, both spouses should be present at meetings.

Are there retirement funds?	Where are they?
	How can they be obtained?
Are there pension accounts?	Do all payments stop if the pensioner dies?

What money will continue to provide for the remaining spouse?
Where are documents stored that contain information about finances?
Which bank is the preferred one? Are there accounts in more than one bank?
What specific name are all the accounts in?
What is your spouse's social security number?
What social security funds will be available for the remaining spouse?
If the family has a family safe, what is the combination?
Who is the family lawyer? Does he have a copy of the will? Contact number?

Any non monetary items should be listed somewhere and the list shared with the spouse or surviving children. Men can have valuable guns, medals, or pieces of equipment. Wives need to know what the value is and how those items should be dealt with. A friend of mine nearly tossed out lucrative stock certificates that were at the bottom of a stack of old newspapers. That was not a good filing system.

Men may not realize that pretty antique bowls can be very valuable. Women tend to have preferences for who will receive items or jewelry when they pass. These preferences may or may not be in a will. It is helpful to write down the lineage or special features of an heirloom while parents accurately remember the details. Going through scrapbooks and naming pictures also falls into this category.

If there is no money, no resources, no retirement funds, the surviving spouse also needs to know that. Life will go on for him or her. Will she need to seek employment? Will she have to sell the house? Will she have to live with family? The anxiety of not knowing the options available in the future can be far worse than knowing the truth.

The idea of planning ahead –as a couple– is what we emphasize. No matter what stage of the illness, foresight prevents unnecessary stress. If planning ahead eliminates even one burden or problem, it's of benefit. If your spouse is healed, consider yourself fortunate; and prepared ahead for the future.

One step in planning ahead may be to find a trusted financial counselor. This may be a financial planner, a business-minded family member, or possibly a trusted volunteer in your church. I realized that I didn't need to be an expert in figuring out my finances, but I did need to find someone who was as good at money matters as I was at caregiving. I found a financial "me".

Anticipating Expenses

We tried to anticipate what our retirement expenses would be by following a budget for several years before and after Dean had retired. I had pared our expenses down to a minimum. I learned how to manage electricity and utilities to get the most services for the least outlay. I also refinanced the house to get the lowest monthly payment on the least rate of interest. Many insurance companies will lower rates for the house and car for seniors with good credit ratings. I had to ask. The better deal was waiting for me to inquire.

The fun expenses were the question mark. How much fun could we afford? The real question should have been: How much fun could Dean tolerate? Each year that I worked our budget, I noticed that as Dean became more incapacitated with the disease, our fun expenditures decreased. We went fewer places and spent very little money on entertainment. We still had fun; we just had it differently. Instead of going to theaters, we rented movies. As Dean's health waned, his naps became his favorite times of the day. We still went out several times a week, but we never traveled very far from home or stayed away long. Many of our fun activities, like the concerts in the park, were free.

Being roughly aware of where money was budgeted helped ease the financial anxiety as the medical expenses increased. I realized that the escalated prescription costs were off-set by savings in other categories. Money forfeited when I quit my job was off-set with early Social Security income. Having the budget was definitely helpful when dealing with the unexpected expenses.

Again, I understand how stressful dealing with the cost of a long term illness can be. Even with Medicare, I had no idea what the final price tag would be for Dean's last four days in a hospital. But, from the financial perspective, I was relieved to learn that once hospice became involved, the care was free. I received no bills for the seven days that Dean was in a coma in a hospice center. That was a huge relief when I was trying to sort through all the money issues after he passed.

One final comment needs to be added to the planning-ahead-suggestion list. Some thought should be given to expenses that will be incurred after a spouse passes. While trying to adjust to the reality that Dean had passed, and recovering from all that had occurred his last week, I woke up one morning and realized that the world had not stopped just because mine had. I was expected to pay all my bills.

If it wasn't sad enough to lose my husband, I also lost all our sources of income. Pensions and social security payments stopped at his death. A few accounts that were in my name continued to pay, but did not contain sufficient funds to cover our bills. Fortunately, Dean had been foresighted in this area as well. There was an account that became available at his death to pay for last expenses, medical expenses and monthly bills until all his accounts could be moved and activated in my name. I had to live from that account for five months until everything started flowing again.

I emphasize strongly that it's better to be prepared and not need it, than to not prepare and end up in a raging storm of financial chaos.

Chapter 15

Preparing Ahead with Legal Issues

Lewy Body Dementia is listed as an incurable disease. Research is working to extend quality of life for those with LBD; but as I write this, the reality is that families need to become prepared for the inevitable.

Dean and I took solace throughout our married years knowing that regardless of who became sick first, the other had all the legal papers in order. Being prepared eased some of the stress and anxieties for both of us. This section is not meant to serve as legal advice. Only definitions of important terms will be offered. Based on my experience, the sooner a family can talk with an attorney the better.

Important Legal Documents

Durable Power of Attorney for Health Care

This is a document that allows a person to authorize another person to make medical decisions for them. Specifically, this would allow the authorized person to make decisions with the doctor should the person be unable to make decisions for himself or herself. The document should be officially prepared by an attorney. The person would need to sign the document with witnesses. As an official document, it should be stored in a safe place for ready access.

Durable Power of Attorney

This document, also prepared by an attorney, authorizes another person to make financial and legal decisions for the person should the person be unable to make decisions for himself or herself. The person would need to sign the document with witnesses. As an official document, it should be stored in a safe place for ready access.

Will

If there's anything good about having a long-term illness, it may be that there's time for everyone to put there personal and business affairs in order. Leaving a will is a loving gesture from one spouse to another. When a person does not leave a will, a court will decide what will happen with any personal funds and property, and take some of those personal funds to make that decision. We used an attorney to make our wills early in our married life. As our life situation changed over the years, we changed the particulars of the will. There will be books in the library that can help in preparing a will.

Living Will Declaration

This is a document that states that the person signing the Living Will wants his family and the medical specialists to honor his wishes not to prolong life by use of artificial means should death be inevitable and should he/she be in a permanently unconscious state or terminal condition.

Do Not Resuscitate (DNR)

This is a different name for the living will. The agent authorized by the person in the durable power of attorney documents can notify the medical team of the patient's end of life preferences. The doctors directing care during the last days are obligated to provide comfort care but not authorized to do extensive medical procedures when the patient has a DNR on the medical chart.

Mayo Clinic has a consumer help page that addresses all of these terms in easy to understand terminology. http://www.mayoclinic.com/health/living-wills/HA00014/

It was not easy to talk to my husband about the end of life decisions, but we did it. When he slipped into a coma, and I needed to be his spokesperson and carry out his wishes; I was prepared. I knew exactly what his wishes were.

Chapter 16

Spiritual Support

A right time to hold on and another to let go,
—Ecclesiastes 3:5 The Message

It is unspeakably difficult to watch as a loved one's strength and vitality drain away during the last days. I began to see significant changes for my husband in June of 2010. He needed three naps a day and twelve hours of sleep at night. He was seeing double most of the time. He might be present with me for a couple hours each day, but most of the time his mind was jumbled. His balance was gone; he needed the wheelchair most of the time.

I wasn't ready to give in to the disease. I wanted miracles. I wanted him to be well. I searched, prayed, and bargained with God to grant some peace with his sickness. I am sharing this desperation because Lewy Body in full force will win. Caregivers may find themselves where I was that summer.

My purpose in this chapter is to encourage others to get overwhelming emotions to the surface. Share the heavy caregiving load to decrease the weight. Finding a source of spiritual support may be what allows a caregiver to persevere with unconditional love.

I mentioned in the chapter on burn-out that I journaled letters to God. When I journaled, I felt an indescribable presence in the letters. The free-association-writing seemed to come alive as if God was sitting beside me writing through my computer keys or my pen. The messages in my letters contained warm, loving, compassionate advice. If I could pick the best father in the world, it would be the sender of the words in my letters.

Because it was such a powerful resource for me, I have chosen to share my bird saga, to illustrate very directly the power within the journal writing.

The Power of a Letter to God

Dear God,

I lay in bed last night, and pondered why the little bird in my front yard was so important to me. I realized I had invested an excessive amount of emotional energy on him every day for two weeks after he fell out of the tree, and had a nest land on top of his head, through no fault of his own. I knew I couldn't change nature and that any day he might not make it. There was very little I could do, except hope and pray.

This morning, Monday, I found the nest empty, no birdie at all. About three feet away, his little body lay flat in the grass. I was sure some animal had mauled him. The natural thing was to praise him for his good fight in overcoming all the odds that were against him.

When I came back a few minutes later to clean up the mess, he was again bouncy alert, gobbling food from the mommy and chirping between bites. The chances of his surviving were incredibly slim, and yet he has been surviving and getting stronger every day.

He has become my mascot for Dean. If the baby bird can make it, maybe Dean can also overcome all his adversities and become well again. I recognize it as a sign that you, God, hold the birds, as well as, all of us in your hands.

To walk outside with Ann this afternoon, at just that five minute window of time was a miracle. As we watched, my birdie rose up from the tall grass, hopped across the uncut lawn, and eventually made it into the neighbor's yard. It was heartwarming to see the mommy fly to him with a huge worm, feed him, and gently coax him into the safe bushes by my neighbor's house. Had I not been present for that tender moment, I would never have known what had happened to him.

This entire adventure with the bird was more amazing than words can express. I thank you for this little bird that you sent to me. And I am thrilled that I was able to witness his safe crossing to freedom today.

It's your turn, God.

Love, Judy

I am glad you enjoyed the baby bird saga. And you interpreted the moral of the story pretty well. You are doing well to remember that all things come together for those who love the Lord. It is only my will whether Dean should be well.

Your personal saga will, indeed, come together. You have more lessons yet to learn. Patience and gentleness are two that come to mind. Remember that I have used nature to teach my lessons since Adam and Eve. He, who seeks, will find.

I will not leave you without support, or give you lessons without a purpose. You need to develop the patience and gentleness for other sagas that you will encounter.

Sleep well, my child.

Love, God

As I journaled, I reflected on the bird drama in my front yard and the outpouring of emotions that the survival of the bird brought to the surface. I was able to identify the fragility of the little bird within Dean. The journal let me dump my negative thoughts into the letter and receive understanding, compassion, and hope. Dean would be taken care of from an Entity far more effective at fixing brokenness than I was.

Through my writing, I knew intuitively, beyond all doubt, that the fragile birdie in my yard was also a symbol for the distraught birdie inside my own soul. But, there was no need to worry; she too was being tended to by an amazing God.

Finding a Spiritual Resource

Journaling may not be an option for everyone reading this book. One friend, who cared for her husband for nine years, joined a support group in her church. On especially bad weeks, she had a group of people who were willing to pray with her, bring in food, or listen. Another friend found a source of strength in support groups organized by local Parkinson Associations in her area. Another turned to other widows because they were able to offer suggestions and extend the compassion that could energize her to continue "for one more day".

Reading can resonate. The Bible is filled with good people who had to endure catastrophic situations. I found several books at the library on caregiving, Alzheimer's, and Dementia that helped me feel a part of a larger circle of sisters.

Our message is to learn to breathe during the day, make time for your entire self: body, mind, and spirit. You will become a better caregiver and companion if you find a well to draw from when your reserves are depleted. No one should do this job without support for the spirit.

And lastly, I hope you will recognize a miracle if/when you receive one. It can be the most powerful source of strength and comfort possible. I offer the following story as just one of many that we experienced.

The Gift

Toward the end of the summer of 2010, it was blatantly obvious that Dean's life was slipping out of my control, and there was nothing I could do. I recall feelings of anguish mixed with apprehension and sadness. I continued to have faith that God was in charge, but my thoughts obsessed with how Dean's final days would go. Could I continue to care for him to the end? Would he have a great deal of pain? Would I be strong enough to support him emotionally? Who would be there to support me emotionally? Was I strong enough to follow through with whatever needed to be done after his passing? My prayers were filled with pleas for help.

In spite of his physical weakness, I honored his request to visit the Football Hall of Fame in Canton, Ohio. He slept on a mattress in the back of my SUV for the four hour trip from Cincinnati to Canton. The next morning he was as excited as a child on Christmas morning. As we toured the museum, he seemed to summon energy from the depths of his being. It was a totally wonderful occasion for him. He inhaled anything that had to do with his favorite football team, the Cleveland Browns, for FOUR hours.

The next day on our way home, we drove into a flash rain storm. The weather changed from blue skies to pelting rain to beautiful blue skies again, within a matter of minutes. As we drove into the sunshine, we saw the largest, most complete rainbow that I had ever seen. Absolutely Spectacular! A gift that only a Godly father could bestow!

That rainbow was filled with confirmations for me: taking Dean on such a strenuous trip WAS a good idea; I would be able to finish our caregiving adventure together; and his passing would be gentle. Most importantly I felt as I watched that rainbow that I wasn't alone and never would be.

I drove the rest of the way home with an assurance that whatever happened, it would be ok. I was able to let go and let God.

Dean slipped into a coma a month later. All of my prayers were answered: I was able to care for him at home until the end; he had a gentle passing at a Hospice facility; and I had an outpouring of support from family and friends.

Caring for my wonderful husband was a noble endeavor. I am honored to be able to share it. He will be missed by many, but we are all better for having shared in his life adventure.

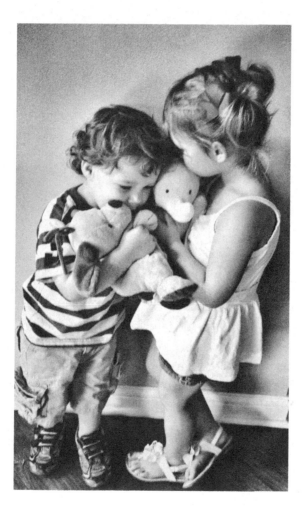

Chapter 17

Afterthoughts

A time for birth and another for death,
—Ecclesiastes 3:2 The Message

It is fitting that this afterthought be offered for care of self after the loved one finishes his journey. I am offering some of the many positive things that helped me get through the first few weeks after my husband died.

Getting through the first days needed a new way of thinking. I was in a valley I had never been in before. It helped to hang Dean's favorite burnt orange shorts on a peg near my bed. Each night I would talk to the shorts and tell them everything that had happened during the day. It was almost like talking to Dean.

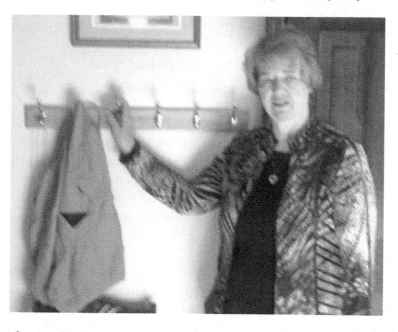

After 'our' talk, I would arrange many pillows around me to simulate his touch in the bed. One of the best pillows was a puppy dog pillow that, somehow, seemed to radiate heat back to me. If I sandwiched it between my back and another pillow, I felt a warm body heat on my back all night.

Setting up the bed for restful sleep seemed to allow my mind to wander into interesting dreams. In one, I was searching for Dean everywhere and couldn't find him. When I woke in the morning and realized that it was a dream, I felt a sense of relief that I wasn't responsible to keep him safe anymore. He was finally safe.

I found that there is a process I had to go through to move away from my life as a dedicated caregiver. I had to follow my own advice in Chapter 3:

Stay positive

Avoid negative thinking by giving myself permission to do what I needed to do

Create new "Moments and Memories"

Utilize coping strategies to help deal with the emotional challenges

Seek quality of life

Extend Permissions to Your Self

Caregivers are allowed to feel a sense of relief.

Caregivers should not feel guilty if they find that they are experiencing a feeling of relief after a loved one finally completes his journey with the disease. I found that my grieving started three years earlier when I accepted that my husband had an incurable disease. I grieved at each new loss of function and each new symptom that forced us to make yet another adjustment. I didn't realize it as I was in the middle of the battle, but I was figuratively holding my breath each day for the last three years of Dean's life. All my efforts worked to make sure that I didn't overlook something, or inadvertently make a misstep that would cause Dean more pain and trauma.

When I finally released him to the Hospice nurses and accepted the fact that Dean would never be coming back home, I was surprised that I experienced a sense of euphoria. I found myself almost silly one morning as I drove around town and ended up getting a relaxing coffee, before I went into the hospice center for my visit.

The euphoric feelings were embarrassing. My husband was in the valley of death, where did the euphoria come from? Close friends and family explained that my sense of relief was centered on the fact that we, Dean and I, had completed a heavy job, and done it extremely well. We had dodged many problems that could have surfaced to make his journey even more painful and incapacitating.

There was definitely a phase of overwhelming relief that the long awaited final act had arrived and had happened with a minimal of pain and suffering for him.

a time for war, and a time for peace.
—Ecclesiastes 3:8 RSV

Caregivers are permitted to make the decisions about the final preparations.

When a caregiver has made every daily decision for the spouse for an extended time, she has the right to make the final decisions regarding his passing. Family may want to help and may have strong opinions with good intentions. After Dean entered hospice, it would have been easy to quit all my caregiving duties. I gave myself permission to stay in charge through all the many hospice decisions.

Because Dean and I had discussed the end of life decisions during his last summer before he went into Hospice, I had confidence that I was carrying out his final wishes. On Monday morning in the hospital, when the doctor confirmed that Dean had gone into a coma, I was able to remind the doctor that Dean had a DNR and did not wish any "treatment" if the coma was indeed terminal. Our doctor immediately agreed with me and suggested that hospice was the best solution at that stage. Knowing full well what Dean's preferences were, I was able to stand strong with the hospice program to discontinue food and water while he was in the coma. I was able to carry out his plan to donate his body to science and to the Lewy Body Dementia research department.

I listened to opinions of friends and family, but I gave myself permission to make all the decisions pertaining to his memorial service. It was an occasion to remember all of Dean's successes in life, and to cheer his choice to live life to the fullest up to the end. It was a celebration of who he was and how deeply he loved his family and his friends. Others told me that they felt Dean would have enjoyed the positive upbeat atmosphere of the service as a way to send him forth. Others might not choose to begin a memorial service with the *Star Spangled Banner* and end the service with *Silent Night*, but I knew Dean would have enjoyed both.

As I look back, I have no regrets about my decisions. That gives me peace.

Accept permission to begin making changes.

Each person will make changes when it feels comfortable to do so. The acceptance of Dean's inevitable passing was easier while I was sitting by his side in the hospice room, than when I was in our house by myself. I wasn't able to get to sleep or stay asleep. For many nights, I would wake thinking that I had heard him call my name. Just walking past his bedroom made me nauseated.

When neighbors asked if I needed help, I took their offer. We completely stripped and gutted everything in the bathroom and bedroom that reminded me of Dean's days of sickness. Curtains, carpeting, bedding were all disposed of. We painted the walls a fresh new color. New carpeting changed the painful memories to hopeful emotions. As soon as I started sleeping in the 'new' bedroom, I began to sleep deeply and restfully.

I found later when I talked to other widows in my church that they also had a need to clean out and clean up. As we purged the physical surroundings, it seemed to clean out the negative memories associated with the disease. We all agreed that it may have been easier to make big decisions because we had been caregivers for many years. Making big changes in our houses almost felt like breathing in new life after a long winter.

Changing the color of the bedroom was just the start. In the year after Dean passed, I ventured out to do many new and different activities. Shopping for groceries felt weird. I needed to buy food differently. The first vacation without him was emotional, but turned out to be filled with wonderful memories. As I write this, I no longer feel compelled to do the routines that I did with Dean. Each week, I have gained an awareness of something new about myself and my interests. It is as if I am making a new friend, and the new friend is me.

Chapter 18

The Valley of Grief

A time to weep, and a time to laugh;
a time to mourn, and a time to dance;
—Ecclesiastes 3:4 RSV

In the early months after Dean passed, I found that I was at a very low
point with my grief. I could function normally during the day at home or
with friends if I acted as if I wasn't a widow. At night all my sleep strategies
failed me. I would lie in bed vacillating between panic and despair. I fought
reliving the memories of our lives together; because I was afraid if I started
to think about the past, I would get stuck there and not be able to travel
back to the present. One night in the dark, I felt like I was standing on
a cliff. Below in a valley was my life with Dean, the good and the ugly. I
knew if I looked into that valley, I would lose control and fall into the
middle of all those memories. I was sure I would start to cry and never be
able to stop.

The next morning, I realized that I needed to find a bridge that
would allow easy access from today to all the yesterdays of the past 40
years. Humor was the bridge. I determined to spend some quiet time
everyday for 30 days and write down at least one funny memory each
day. At first nothing came. Then the incidents began to wash over my
mind. As I wrote them down, I wanted more and more. Humor not only
became the bridge to transport me easily from the past to the present, it

became the plaster to patch up the holes in my heart. I bought a plaque to hang in my newly painted and decorated bathroom that equated laughter with music in the heart. Each morning it reminds me to be open to the humor in our everyday happenings.

As I shared some of the stories that I remembered with friends and family, they also began to remember and share new stories with me. As we retold the stories, we laughed again and created a new laugh memory out of an old story. Humor became the balm we all needed to ease the pain so we could share the joy of Dean's real personality. His smile, his laugh, and his witty reaction to a goofy incident were all pebbles that he dropped into my heart for 40 years. The expanding ripples continue to gently wash over my soul and bring ever more smiles to my face. As my son recalls, "Dad was a funny guy!" That part of his personality brought me joy in our marriage and now will live on in my memories.

Grief is Personal

We have the right to move through the grief stages in our own personal way. Hopefully all caregivers will realize that grieving is a process. Each person will need to grieve as best fits his or her own needs. It is not something that can be wished away. The pain must be felt and the loss eventually acknowledged before life can return to some different form of normal.

I have never been one to cry easily around other people. My family was almost offended when I was not crying continually during Dean's days in hospice. I did my tears privately and was comfortable comforting other people and staying calm and efficient. I would have been wrong if I had expected everyone else in the family to react as I was able to do, both immediately and after several months. I gave them permission to grieve their way. I expected them to allow me to do what I needed to do. When my son suggested that I immediately sell the house and move closer to him, I was able to say no to any big decisions for at least a year.

Thoughts to Ponder When Moving Through the Tunnel of Grief

In one LBD support meeting, the counselors encouraged us to work through our grief by talking about the loved one any possible chance. I found that to be true. I gained comfort by talking about Dean at outings. It is truly energizing and liberating to hear people's heartfelt stories about their experiences with him.

When our grandchildren came to visit, we talked about Grampa. The conversations usually started with how sad they were that Grampa wasn't with us to play. They always ended with "Remember When" stories. I would ask them if they remembered how much fun we had on their visits. Did they remember jumping into bed with him in the mornings to wake him up? Did they remember the funny critters he would make with our playdoh sessions? Did they remember how he would tickle them and how hard they would laugh? For them as for me, remembering the moments of joy and laughter bridged the valley of our grief.

I hope for two things as I finish this discussion about grief. First, I hope I create many valuable memory moments with my grandchildren over the next twenty years. Secondly, when they enter into the tunnel of grief at my passing, I hope they take the time to play "Remember When" with each other so that all those memories we made together will stay ever fresh in their minds.

Widowhood Is More Than a Label; It Is a Journey.

As I finish this book, I have been able to reflect back over the past year since Dean passed. I realize that I have grown, I am not the same person I was. It took only one second for me to move into the category labeled "widow". It took several days, tears, compassionate gestures, observations, and courageous decisions to appreciate the experience of being a widow. I offer these insights to you, my dear readers, as a gift, a symbolic rainbow. May my observations about my journey into the experience of widowhood, reveal the same full magnificent symbol of hope that I experienced on the road home with Dean in the back seat. The storm doesn't have to last forever.

I am more than my parenting years, my married years, and my caregiving years. Experiencing the transition of life to death has made me more alive. Receiving the bounty of compassion from friends and family has made me more outwardly focused. Carrying the cross of caregiving through the five years of fire, has given me a confidence to do whatever God has planned for me to do next. I fully expect to have setbacks in the years to come and eventually medical challenges of my own. After completing the extremely difficult task of taking care of my ailing husband, I am fully assured of two things. Nothing can be more difficult to do than what I have already done; and God will always be there to guide me through it.

Enduring Stage

As I look back to observe the changes over the past year, I recognize a metamorphosis. At first being a widow had to be endured. It took great effort to get through a 24 hour day, to make all the decisions, to see into the future. I endured the first two weeks by staying extremely busy. Revamping the house to make it a pleasant place for me to live helped. Organizing Dean's memorial service with a slide show and picture posters of all the stages of his life was comforting. Each night for those two weeks I would drop into bed absolutely bone tired.

Getting away to help my son and his family move to a new city gave me purpose and took my mind off of everything. When I returned to my home after five weeks, I was past the enduring stage and ready to move into what ever needed to happen next.

Experience Stage

After months of home neglect, I was ready to start reorganizing my life. That included sorting through a mound of bills. I don't recommend attempting that project to the faint hearted. Some of the bills were shockingly high. After the rest and revitalization with family, I was able to determine which bills were warranted and which contained errors. I was up to the task.

The first time I mentioned being a widow, I was complaining to a customer service representative about an overcharge on a bill. That was the first time I let myself acknowledge and experience widowhood. To admit that I was a widow meant that I had to admit that Dean wasn't just visiting his mother. He really wasn't coming back. I had to take charge of my own life.

When the representative's demeanor changed on the phone, my metamorphosis moved to a new awareness. As she applied a credit to my bill and told me how sorry she was for my loss, I realized that it was not going to be easy, but I could do it. Sometimes I chose to share and sometimes I chose not to mention that I was widowed. As I began to experience all the changes that I had to face as a single, I realized that I was beginning to look at my status from an adventure attitude. Being a widow had a full range of new things to experience, not all were painful and sad. It was sort of like trying on a new coat to see how it fit.

The Journey Can be Embraced.

I have finally arrived at a mental place where I accept my aloneness. This does not diminish the love I have for my husband. Quite the contrary, I still occasionally talk to his shorts at night, but now all the positive memories of our life together are easily remembered and do not cause me pain.

He finished his life-book and did it in an honorable way. To want him back would be wishing for him to go through his exit journey again. He was able to be upbeat with all aspects of a nasty disease. I finally realized that I needed to become positive minded about my life as a widow. The ability to let him go and to give myself permission to move on happened by degrees, but I am now at a place where a better way to honor him is to make the most of the time I have left.

I am beginning to wake up in the morning and embrace this beginning to the next chapter in my life. I am free to make it as interesting as I choose. I can learn to line-dance. I can travel the world. I can write books, meet new people, and join new organizations. I didn't seek widowhood, but since I now am in it, I realize that I should follow Dean's example and play the hand that I have been dealt, expecting to win.

And at some point down the road, may others say of me that I chose to *Dance*.

APPENDIX 1
TIME LINE

Time Line for Dean Jennings's LBD Symptoms

Disease Progression	Anxiety but no Physical Symptoms					
Year and life status	Symptom	Diagnosis	Ambulation	Level of Care	Medication	Modifications in Live Style
2003	Anxiety	None	Competitive tennis	Fully independent	Cialis	None
Employed	Forgetfulness		Running	Stage 0		
	Sleepiness					
	Gained 35 lbs					
	Minimal Symptoms	Early				
2004	Less Anxiety	None	Tennis	Independent	Cialis	
Retired	Forgetful		Hamstring muscles hurting	Entered Stage 1		
House keeping	Sleepiness Continues			Mild health issues		
Shopping groceries	Posture, less erect		Fell bicycle riding			
Stage	Minimal Disability	Early				
2005	"Stumbilitis"	Mayo Clinic		Independent		Less housekeeping duties expected
Sleeps a lot	Feet heavy	? PD		Some serious	Cialis	
	Hamstring pain	HS strain		health issue	Muscle relaxers	
	Sleepy			suspected		
	Whispery voice	Broke collar bone	Fell on court	Stage 1		
Stage	Minimal Disability		Almost No Symptoms			

Time Line for D Jennings's LBD Symptoms pg 2

Year and life status	Symptom	Diagnosis	Ambulation	Level of Care	Medication	Modifications in Live Style
2006	Min. stumbling	Aring	Good tennis	Independent	Sinemet	None
Exercise in	Voice good	Neurology	1.5 hours	Good as new	Cialis	
PT clinic	HS healed	PD		Stage 0		
Cruise	Occ. Hand twitching			Before Cruise		
	Poor tol heat					
	Dropsie with hands					
After cruise	Serious sleep problems			Stage 1 After Cruise		
Stage	Moderate Disability	Middle				
2007	Rash on face	PD	Tennis			Stopped Night driving
	Smell ↓		30 minutes		Sinemet	
House keeping	Anxiety ↑		Walking good	Independent	Anxiety pill Paxil	
and home	Depressed		Exercising Daily	But slow	Cialis	
alone	Constipation !		Poor foot sensation		Miralax Daily	
	Problem Solving ↓		Poor coordination			
			Shower chair			
Stage	Moderate					
2008 Spring	Sleep good	PD	Walking good	Independent	Tylenol PM	
	Memory poor		Exercising Daily	Slow		
	Handwriting ↓					
Stage	Severe					
2008			Balance Poor			
	Seizures		Would fall			Stopped all driving

Summer	Hallucinations	LBD	Without support	1 week of constant care	Excelon for dementia	Walker or cane before drug. Running after
	Pass out		Walker		Mididrine	
Stage	**3 Moderate**					
Fall	Hallucinations under control		Running	Independent		Planned Mediterranean Cruise
						Walks around neighborhood by self

Time Line for D Jennings's LBD Symptoms pg 3

Year and life status	Symptom	Diagnosis	Ambulation	Level of Care	Medication	Modifications in Live Style
Stage	**Hospital after Drug Reaction**					
2009	Violent Hallucinations	LBD, Drug reaction	None	100%	Violent reaction to urinary pill	Invalid, hospital bed, Assistance with all activities 24 hours a day
Spring	No balance	Urinary tract infection			Antibiotic	Judy home. Full demential
Hospital	Flailing arms, incoherent	Sinus infect				
Stage	**Moderate,Severe**					
Cruise May	Knee buckling					In wheelchair by end of summer all time
Summer	Incontinent	LBD	Walker long distances	Help for showers	Sinemet, Excelon	Many dependent days
	Sleepy				Paxil Namenda	More help needed for care
Stage	**Moderate**					
2009	Miraculous	LBD	Walking well with cane	Minimal help needed	Sinemet, Excelon	Health returned, Back to level of abilities of 18 months before.

Year and life status	Symptom	Diagnosis	Ambulation	Level of Care	Medication	Modifications in Live Style
Fall	Recovery in	Sinus infect			Paxil Namenda	No driving or tennis but all else mostly indep
	response to		Walker long distances	Help for showers		Occasionally a bad couple of days
	divine interaction		Balance good			
	Memory good		No tennis			
Stage	Varies: Moderate Severe Totally Dependent					
2010		Sinus infect				
Jan-Apr	Periods of mental confusion	LBD	Walked stairs during flood ordeal	Daily care assistance	Same	Easy to manage till flood, then much more dependent
	Arm support when walking	LBD				
May to Aug	Total Care		Wheelchair mostly, after flood	Many days of total care	same	Invalid, Many naps,
	All symptoms. Total care all of the time				Seroquel	In bed for night at 7:30, 2-3 naps a day
	Dementia part of every day					
Sept		LBD	Dif standing	Many days in bed		
	Pain in back, joints, eyes		Max Assist to transfer	Bed baths		Invalid almost all of the time. Exercised as able. Walked chair to chair as able
29-Sep	Rolled out of bed and no ability to bear weight		Not able to bear wt			Hospital for tests. LBD had advanced

Year and life status	Symptom	Diagnosis	Ambulation	Level of Care	Medication	Modifications in Live Style
4-Oct	Coma in hosp					Transferred to hospice
10-Oct	Died Peacefully					

APPENDIX 2
PARKINSON-PLUS-SYNDROMES

as referenced by Arif Dalvi MD and Stephen M. Bloomfield MD[4]

Multiple System Atrophy

Progressive Supranuclear Palsy

Parkinsonism-Dementia-ALS Complex

Corticobasal Ganglionic Degeneration

Diffuse Lewy Body Disease *

*Other sources label this syndrome as Lewy Body Dementia, Lewy Body Disease, Parkinson's Disease with Dementia, and Dementia with Lewy Bodies, Cortical Lewy Body Disease, Lewy Body Variant of Alzheimers's

REFERENCES

1. National Family Caregivers Association. Available at https://www.thefamilycaregiver.org/who_are_family_caregivers/care_giving_statstics.cfm#1

   Accessed June 6, 2012

2. Lieberman, Abraham. <u>Shaking up Parkinson Disease, Fighting like a Tiger, Thinking Like a Fox.</u>

   Jones and Bartlett Publishers, Massachusetts. 2002, p 196.

3. Shriver, Maria. <u>Alzheimer's Disease in America.</u> Free Press, Division of Simon and Schuster, NY. 2010 Intro.

4. Dalvi A, Bloomfield S. Parkinson-Plus-Syndromes. eMedicine Neurology. August 27, 2008

5. Mayo Clinics. Rochester, NY; Jacksonville, FL; Phoenix, AZ. www.mayoclinic.com

6. Aring Neurology, UC Physicians. Cincinnati, Ohio.

7. National Parkinson's Foundation. What is Parkinson's Disease? www.parkinson.org Accessed June 6, 2012

8. Parkinson's Disease Foundation. What is Parkinson's Disease? www.pdf.org Accessed June 6, 2012

9. Lewy Body Dementia Association. What is LBD? www.lbda.org Accessed June 6, 2012

10. Alzheimer's Association. Life with Alz. www.alz.org Accessed June 6, 2012

11. Lieberman A, McCall, M. <u>100 Questions and Answers about Parkinson Disease</u>, Jones and Bartlett Publishers, Mass., 2003,

12. Giroux, M, Farris, S. <u>Every Victory Counts</u>. Davis Phinney Foundation for Parkinson's Sunflower Seminars, Cincinnati, Ohio, 2010.

13. Brown, Dorian. Relearning Kinesia Treatment for Parkinson's Disease and Related Movement Disorders. Seminar, Cross Country Education 2010.

14. Whitworth, Helen Buell, Whitworth J. <u>A Caregiver's Guide to Lewy Body Dementia</u>. demosHEALTH. New York. 2011.

15. Hohen and Yahr Staging Scale, http://neurosurgery.mgh.harvard.edu/Functional/pdstages.htm

16. Unified Parkinson Disease Rating Scale (UPDRS) http://neurosurgery.mgh.harvard.edu/Functional/pdstages.htm

17. Medline Plus, U.S. National Library of Medicine, Hallucinations, www.nlm.nih.gov/medlineplus/ency/article/003258.htm Accessed June 6, 2012

18. 1 Evanovitch, Janet. Stephanie Plum Novel series. St Martin's Press,. New York, N Y.

19. Rabens, Nancy Mace. <u>The 36 Hour Day</u>. Johns Hopkins University Press. Maryland. 2006.

20. Josh Groban, *Awake*, Nov 2006, Reprise Records

21. White, DK, Wagenaar RC, Ellis TD, Tickle-Degnen L. Changes in walking activity and endurance following rehabilitation for people with Parkinson disease. Arch Phys Med Rehabil. 2009 Jan:90(1):43-50.

22. Ridgel AL, Vitek JL, Alberts JL. Forced, Not Voluntary, Exercise Improves Motor Function in Parkinson's Disease Patients. Neurorehabil Neural Repair 2009; 23; 600.

23. Fuzhong Li, Harmer P, Fitzgerald K, Eckstrom E, Stock R, Galver J, Maddalozzo G, Batya, S. Tai Chi and Postural Stability in Patients with Parkinson Disease. N Engl J Med, 2012, 366:511-519.

24. Garth Brooks. *The Dance*. Written by Tony Arata, Produced by Allen Reynolds, Liberty Records, 1995.

25. Nikken, Inc., Irvine, CA, www.nikken.com

26. Robinson DS. Anticholinergic Effects of Drugs and Cognition in the Elderly. Primary Psychiatry. 2009. 16(5): 19-21.

27. Lewy Body Dementia Association, An Introduction to LBD, Understanding LBD, Symptoms and Treatments. www.lbda.org Accessed June 6, 2012

28. Waugh, Diana., <u>I Was Thinking</u>, Conversation Starters to Use with Loved Ones with Cognitive Loss. 2008. dwaugh@accesstoledo.com. ISBN 978-1-4357-1051-1

29. Hannaford, Carla <u>Awaking the Child Heart</u>, Jamilla Nur Publishing, Hawaii, 2002,

30. Bible, Psalm 23:5, King James Version

31. Mayo Clinic Consumer Health In-depth, http://www.mayoclinic.com/health/living-wills/HA00014/

INDEX

INFORMATION ABOUT THE AUTHOR

Judy Towne Jennings, PT, MA is a physical therapist. She was an enthusiastic baby development specialist until caring for her husband forced her to become an expert in caregiving for Lewy Body Dementia.

Judy has always been an advocate, a voice for those who could not speak for themselves. She has lectured extensively on the importance of early tummy time for infants to assure that they attain developmental milestones. What babies do in the first six weeks and six months impacts how they will do in preschool and later in school. Information on baby development and the importance of tummy time for infants is available on her website www.fit-baby.com.

With the experience gained while caring for her husband, she will now become a voice for those with a deteriorating neurological disease. Lewy Body Dementia is still not well known, and few understand the course of the disease. It is heartbreaking to see a person with LBD in a nursing facility suffering from the errant administration of drugs. It is sad to see the interaction of families with someone who has less skills one day than the day before. The patient is accused of being lazy, stubborn, oppositional; when in fact mental and physical skills come and go without any control.

Judy will be available to lecture about her caregiving experiences and her book. She can be reached through her website.

Judy lives in the Cincinnati area. She loves to spend time with her family and continues to play tennis, do research, and travel.

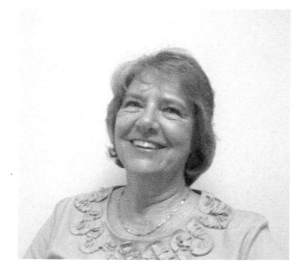

Made in the USA
Coppell, TX
04 May 2021